SUFFERING THE SILENCE

CHRONIC LYME DISEASE IN AN AGE OF DENIAL

ALLIE CASHEL

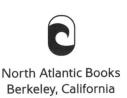

North Atlantic Books
Berkeley, California

Published by
North Atlantic Books
Berkeley, California

Cover photo © Steve Buckley/Shutterstock.com
Author photo © Lily Colman, www.lilycolman.com.
Cover and book design by John Yates at Stealworks.com
Printed in the United States of America

Suffering the Silence: Chronic Lyme Disease in an Age of Denial is sponsored and published by the Society for the Study of Native Arts and Sciences (dba North Atlantic Books), an educational nonprofit based in Berkeley, California, that collaborates with partners to develop cross-cultural perspectives, nurture holistic views of art, science, the humanities, and healing, and seed personal and global transformation by publishing work on the relationship of body, spirit, and nature.

North Atlantic Books' publications are available through most bookstores. For further information, visit our website at www.northatlanticbooks.com or call 800-733-3000.

The following information is intended for general information purposes only. Individuals should always see their health care provider before administering any suggestions made in this book. Any application of the material set forth in the following pages is at the reader's discretion and is his or her sole responsibility.

Library of Congress Cataloging-in-Publication Data

Cashel, Allie.
  Suffering the silence : chronic Lyme disease in an age of denial / Allie Cashel.
    pages cm
  Summary: "A young sufferer of chronic Lyme disease investigates the roots of the illness and the controversy around its acceptance as a chronic illness; features the stories of chronic Lyme patients from around the world and their struggle for recognition and treatment."-- Provided by publisher.
  Includes bibliographical references.
  ISBN 978-1-58394-924-5 (trade paperback) -- ISBN 978-1-58394-925-2 (e-book)
  1. Lyme disease--Patients--Biography. 2. Chronically ill--Biography. 3. Cashel, Allie. 4. Lyme disease--Social aspects. 5. Lyme disease--Psychological aspects. 6. Chronic diseases--Social aspects. 7. Chronic diseases--Psychological aspects. 8. Denial (Psychology)--Social aspects. 9. Stigma (Social psychology) I. Title.
  RC155.5.C37 2015
  616.9'246--dc23
                                                          2015002660

1 2 3 4 5 6 7 8 SHERIDAN 19 18 17 16 15

Printed on recycled paper.

CONTENTS

FOREWORD BY DR. BERNARD RAXLEN

Virgil is credited with stating: "Felix qui potuit rerum cognoscere causas," or, "fortunate is he who knows the causes of things."

In this book Allie Cashel, a longtime patient of mine, has conducted her own intelligently written, deeply moving inquiry into "the causes of things"—in this case, the various causes of the multitude of effects of chronic Lyme disease.

This is an unflinchingly honest story of self-examination. It is both a starkly unvarnished account of her inner world as well as a poignant history of the physical and emotional pain endured throughout a chronic relapsing disease. Along the way she experienced bewildering, incomprehensible, debilitating symptoms of illness interwoven with periods of elusive, seductive wellness. I say "incomprehensible" because opinions regarding correct diagnoses and proper treatment for her illness swirl in controversy, and she and her family were forced to choose between opposed schools of thought. In this book she chronicles the bitter, intractable debate surrounding chronic Lyme disease, as well as her experience as a patient caught in the crossfire of the antagonists' sometimes brutal assaults.

As a doctor myself, I feel it keenly that the greatest pain Allie's experience brought her came from the hands of other doctors. Unfortunately, physician specialists, ignorant of the basic principles of psychiatry, use completely erroneous misconceptions of psychiatric illness to explain away some patients' chronic debilitated conditions. Although psychiatric illness can arise from tick-borne disease, it is not a root cause, not "the cause of things." With such misdiagnoses the patients' falsely labeled illness gets buried alive in the medical system's "diagnostic graveyard." The subsequent tombstones could have many inscriptions: somatoform disorder, chronic fatigue syndrome, bipolar disorder, ADHD, persistent chronic anxiety, body image distortion, depression, persistent stress disorders, CIFIDS, medically unexplained symptoms . . . the list goes on.

Not surprisingly, the bewildered patients who are victims of "death by diagnosis" come to seriously doubt the reality of their medical condition. The final shovelful of dirt thrown on the coffin comes when the patient is finally told, "It's all in your head." Allie was dealt this blow; the false label attached to her was "psychiatric illness." She beautifully describes how she and her family got swept up in the maelstrom of misdiagnosis: a misunderstanding perpetrated by specialists we are meant to trust.

The denial of tick-borne illness is supported and maintained by an elaborate hierarchy of official misinformation. Laboratory testing is often inadequate or completely misleading. As seronegative Lyme disease is denied by insurance companies, patients who have negative blood test results won't be offered treatment. Sensitive results by specialty labs are ignored or even denigrated. Positive tests are often interpreted as false positive. Sophisticated new culture tests—demonstrating *Borrelia* bacteria grown under special incubated conditions can be identified by monoclonal antibiotic detection—are considered unacceptable by the CDC. Worst of all, the IDSA guidelines, which do not recognize the existence of chronic Lyme disease, and recommend only minimal treatment, are dangerously inadequate. Unfortunately, these outdated guidelines are still used by infectious disease specialists to diagnose and treat Lyme, as well as by other specialists in neurology and rheumatology. And, on the strength of those guidelines, every day insurance companies deny patients coverage they desperately need.

This medical shortsightedness, this refusal to review new important studies on Lyme, is sadly pervasive. Journals, from which physicians draw up-to-date knowledge, are highly selective: they publish only research and opinion articles that support the CDC position on this disease. Allie eloquently describes all of these situations, putting word to the whole complex "denial system" that keeps medical wisdom in stasis, insurance coffers full, and patients' lives drained. This is a system we must work together to overcome.

Though throughout this book Allie draws on her personal experience, what is perhaps most important is that her story is not unique to her—and nor is her suffering. Allie augments her tale with transcripts from interviews she conducted with others suffering from chronic Lyme: interviews that are as poignant as they are authentic. With the undeniable consistency of their experience, they serve to expand readers' understanding of what it means to "suffer the silence" when afflicted with the physical, emotional, and spiritual heartbreak of Lyme disease.

Happily, this book documents the incredible journey that Allie and her fellow patients have survived, offering within these pages a sensitive rendering of the adolescent identity problems and complex family dynamics that can occur under the pressure of chronic relapsing illness. As it is a thoroughly researched treatise on the devastating effects of tick-borne infections, this work's insights will be of special benefit to misunderstood patients newly caught in their own maelstroms of misdiagnosis—especially in learning they are not alone.

There is a sad ironic coincidence to the timing of this introduction. I finished my first draft on the night of November 17, 2014, the very night of the death, at the age of eighty-two, of Dr. William Burgdorfer. As eminent bacteriologist and medical research scientist, and discoverer of the *Borrelia* spirochete that bears his name, Dr. Burgdorfer will most certainly be included in the pantheon of great men and women whose contributions have changed the course of medical history—and by extension uplifted all of humanity.

"We stand on the shoulders of medical giants," is often quoted by physicians. I could never have helped thousands of patients like Allie Cashel without the great work of Dr. Burgdorfer. Patients such as Allie Cashel, and her triumph over Lyme disease, will remain his legacy.

Dr. Bernard Raxlen

PART I

THE ACHES AND PAINS OF DAILY LIVING

Lyme disease *(Lyme borreliosis)* afflicts millions of people worldwide. It is transmitted via the bacterium *Borrelia burgdorferi*, transferred to humans and other mammals through the bites of infected blacklegged ticks. The "standard" symptoms of Lyme disease include headache, fever, joint stiffness, and the infamous bull's-eye rash. For 80 to 90 percent of infected individuals, the disease is manageable, sufficiently treated by the two to six weeks of antibiotic therapy recommended by both the Infectious Disease Society of America and the Centers for Disease Control. But 10 to 20 percent of those afflicted experience a significantly more debilitating litany of symptoms, for an often extended period of time. In these cases, the treatment covered by health insurance is insufficient. Though crippling symptoms persist, the doctors who cannot or choose not to diagnose their condition often explain away unnerving persistent symptoms as the "aches and pains of daily living." This dismissive approach can leave those suffering without an advocate—at the time of perhaps their most desperate need. As a result they are forced to live shadow lives, plagued with disabling symptoms and yet often dismissed by the medical community and by our society as being mentally, rather than physically, ill.

All this from the bite of one tick.

CHAPTER 1

SPINNING OUT OF CONTROL

It started in June of 1998. I was seven years old. At our home in New York, my younger brother Conor and I were outside in the sun, playing some silly game that involved ripping grass from the ground to cover each other's legs. I remember laughing amidst showers of green when suddenly the game changed. Instead of burying me, Conor started clearing the grass off my legs with a determination I didn't understand. Frustrated by this rule change, I tried to clear his legs too, but he stopped me, pointing to a large red rash on the side of my thigh, an angry red circle with a swollen center. Though we didn't speak, we both understood that our game was over.

Within a week I found myself sitting on a leather couch in a doctor's waiting room with my younger siblings. Four of us sat in a row on the couch, with the youngest—still only a few months old, parked in his stroller next to us—completing the line. There was a big teddy bear staring at us from the other side of the room. He wore a lime green T-shirt that had a picture of a bug, crossed-out like a No Smoking sign; I remember wondering what kind of bug that teddy bear didn't want around. I looked at the bear, still and lifeless, and imagined him covered in those little bugs, as though they were a surging, living blanket. I then looked down at the Magic Marker tracing of my rash, a reminder of the bull's-eye that had faded days before. The only proof of its existence was the red circle drawn onto my thigh, retraced every night before bed.

My siblings and I were all given blood tests. Back in the waiting room, I asked the receptionist what kind of bug was on the bear. "It's a deer tick," she told me, as she casually held the door open for a man and his wife. The man carried the woman through the door; her head kept falling away from his shoulder as if she were too weak to hold it up. Her veins showed through her skin, and she was so thin I could see her bones through the clothes hanging off her body. The receptionist just smiled as though everything was normal.

The man placed the woman, limp, into a chair across the room. I remember looking away but then looking back, focusing again on her, waiting to see if she would move or smile, but our parents pushed us out the door before I could see if she came to life.

It's been sixteen years now since that day. I miss the time before then, when the words "Lyme disease" were still relatively meaningless to me.

Following that doctor visit in the summer of 1998, three of my siblings and I were diagnosed with Lyme, a disease that was already part of my family's vernacular, as the same doctor, Dr. Bernard Raxlen, had diagnosed my father with Lyme only a few months earlier.

After our diagnoses, my siblings and I completed the standard course of six weeks of antibiotics. My father had also completed his. By almost all medical standards we were cured, but our bodies insisted on playing devil's advocate.

Ten years later, I fell in love in the spring of 2008 and forgot I had ever felt pain. The parts of my body that had always been heavy suddenly felt light, and everything that was once difficult for me, was now easy. When my father accepted a job in Boston that June, our move didn't fully resonate with me until we started packing up our home. Relocating a family of seven is no easy task, so the focus was not on me when I dented the car, or forgot what I'd done the previous day.

By that time, Lyme disease was something I thought I knew very well. I knew the type of pain it caused. I knew the weight of the fatigue on my limbs and my chest. But something different was happening that fall, something frightening and unfamiliar. On the surface, I was more of a teenager than I ever had been—a seemingly healthy chatterbox who spent too much time at her boyfriend's house. In reality, my mind was starting to go, but no one seemed to notice.

I once imagined losing my mind as a glamorous, controlled descent into darkness. But missing memories, thoughts, or speech—that was never part of my fantasy. It turns out that there's nothing enchanting about surrendering the precious contents of one's consciousness. When you forget something, it disappears from your awareness, and only occasionally does it leave a reminder of its existence. I was a camp counselor that summer, and when I forgot what camper I was supposed to pick up next on my bus route each morning, I wouldn't remember that I had also forgotten the day before. Memories of those forgotten moments never formed. I don't remember singular misfires; I only remember what it felt like when things started spinning out of control.

In early August 2008, my family moved to Hingham, Massachusetts, a town twenty-five minutes outside Boston. As this move necessitated going to a new school for my senior year, we decided it would be best for me to stay in New York to finish high school. I'd live in our house with a family friend—a friend of a friend who I hadn't met actually—until it sold; and in the meantime I'd join them in Massachusetts whenever possible. In mid-August we traveled to Logan International Airport to meet Heather, my house companion for the upcoming school year. A week later Heather and I drove back to Katonah, making small talk about the Spice Girls while I panicked about my decision to leave my family and live with a stranger in an empty house, where my voice echoed if I spoke too loudly. Then, on August 20 I drove my boyfriend, Calvin, to Poughkeepsie for his first year at Vassar College. Back in Katonah that night, I fell asleep wearing his clothes, dreaming of ways to bring everyone together again.

At the time I didn't consider that all these changes could have a damaging effect on my psyche. I just worried about my mom's reaction to my decision to stay in New York, about Heather feeling well-adjusted, or about Calvin's first few weeks at college. I didn't notice that my joints had started to swell, or how often I dropped my pencil. I was genuinely surprised when I was later asked how many car accidents I'd been in that fall, or when exactly I'd started writing reminders about what classes I'd attended each day at school. I didn't understand what was happening to me when I started to notice the words tangling together inside of my sentences.

Lyme sufferers often describe experiencing emerging neurological symptoms as a descent into a dark brain fog. Though my consciousness did feel cloudy, the overwhelming sensation for me was of electrical malfunction. I imagined synapses in my brain as snapped wires along which my thoughts and impulses short-circuited, buzzing and sparking with the frustration of yet another failed connection. Words caught in my throat awaiting their marching orders as I struggled to form the simplest phrases, each word requiring a separate message from the faulty wiring that was my brain.

In hindsight, I realize that I'd been displaying symptoms of neurological dysfunction long before those symptoms were ever named. At my job at the day camp that summer, I struggled with routine tasks that other counselors seamlessly maintained. I carried the daily schedule in my back pocket as a reminder of where I needed to be even though my routine never changed. My campers wore their nametags for two weeks longer than their peers. And while I should have been able to work a full

6

day without pain, at the end of each day that summer I was crippled with exhaustion, aware of every bone in my feet and every fiber in my muscles. During the month of August I was in six minor car accidents, one on the moving-day drive to Massachusetts. To myself and to my family, I blamed all these mishaps on the sun, on being out of shape, on not getting enough sleep. Everything that seemed strange had an obvious, mundane answer, any discrepancy easily explained away.

Though I pretended there was no unsettling root cause behind all these oddities, with each new aberration I was overpowered by fear. At times I could taste it on my tongue, feel it constricting my chest, tightening my breath. The fear was so consuming I didn't give much thought to how these strange developments were affecting the people around me.

The human brain utilizes up to one hundred billion neurons; the speed at which they normally transmit messages makes thoughts feel immediate, even timeless. But in my ravaged condition, I could almost palpably feel my brain misfire. I was hyperaware of each crackling short circuit of each slowly forming thought. Everyone could see that something was wrong, but I couldn't begin to explain what I was experiencing. It was impossible to articulate the bizarre sensations wreaking havoc in my body and brain. Though my family and I had previously dealt with my physical illness, to the point such had become routine, what we experienced that summer left us confused, scared, and flailing. We desperately needed help.

CHAPTER 2

THE DEBATE OVER CHRONIC LYME

The medical and scientific community agree that *Borrelia burgdorferi* is a spirochete bacterium that infects mammals with what we call Lyme disease. The bacterium can be transmitted through the bite of the black-legged tick, which is no bigger than the head of a pin. Because of its size, and since it releases numbing agents and antihistamines before it bites, the tick often goes unnoticed until it's already started the feeding process and latched onto the skin. If the tick is mature and infected with *Borrelia burgdorferi*, it transmits the bacterium as it feeds. If the tick carries any other bacteria, often called co-infections, those bacteria may get transmitted in the same bite. If the patient develops the infamous bull's-eye rash and presents flu-like symptoms, then that patient is infected and should be treated with antibiotics to kill the bacteria, regardless of the test result.

The preceding encompasses the extent of the general agreement about Lyme disease. All other characteristics and questions surrounding Lyme are remarkably divisive; the medical community is split down the middle on issues like diagnosis, treatment, and persistence of infection. As a result, there is no definitive information available on various important details concerning the disease, a modern-day medical phenomenon that, according to current tabulation standards, affects at least 300,000 new people per year in the United States alone. In this book's Appendix C, a chart differentiates the statements and sources regarding a number of these important details, highlighting the sometimes extreme variation among published statements.

The International Lyme and Associated Diseases Society (ILADS) posits that Lyme infection occurs as the tick transmits the bacterium to the mammalian host in its first blood meal. This transmission of the pathogen can occur in a matter of minutes, not hours, days, or weeks, as is often suggested. Early-onset Lyme symptoms, often called "early-localized infection," normally manifest in the body for one to four weeks after the bite.

As for the bull's-eye rash, more accurately called *erythema migrans:* since it's a sure sign of infection—the outside circumference of the bull's-eye actually contains the bacterium—the rash can be a blessing, as it ensures treatment. If treated early and properly, Lyme patients have an excellent chance for complete recovery with no further complications.

But, despite the rash's reputation, only about one-third of people infected with these bacteria present the rash. In fact, two-thirds of those infected never present with the bull's-eye rash, and often they don't even know they're sick. Though they may experience fatigue, achiness, joint pain, fever, and chills, these symptoms are often mistaken for stress or flu—thus, these patients are not treated aggressively, or perhaps not at all. If left untreated, the infection may lie dormant for weeks, months, even years before manifesting more debilitating symptoms. Pain creeps into the muscles of the infected, who may experience weakness and numbness in their extremities. Headaches, described as a tight helmet squeezing the skull, become more frequent. Neurological symptoms may present at this stage, patients perhaps having difficulty sleeping, concentrating, or retaining short-term memories. They can feel besieged: their lives changing without their knowing why.

The advanced forms of tick-borne diseases are called many names.

Late, persistent infection; post-treatment Lyme syndrome; MSIDS; and chronic systemic Lyme disease. This is the most debilitating form of the disease, and also the most contested. Months or years after infection, even if they've received treatment, patients can lose complete control over their bodies. Some develop a disorienting form of neurocognitive dysfunction called *Lyme encephalopathis;* those afflicted can get lost on their way home, can struggle to read, to speak, to hold a fork at dinnertime. Some patients suffer from cardiovascular issues; others must reckon with recurring full-body seizures. Every patient presents symptoms differently in this stage of the disease, which is one of the many reasons it's so hard to diagnose and to treat.

As I mentioned earlier, ticks can carry a number of bacteria; to date, scientists have discovered more than a dozen tick-borne illnesses, any of which can get transmitted with the Lyme bacterium in a single bite. Three seem to appear alongside Lyme more than others: *Babesia, Ehrlichiosis,* and *Bartonella. Babesia* is a malaria-like disease that attacks red blood cells. *Ehrlichiosis* attacks white blood cells in the immune system. As for *Bartonella,* its influence on the body's cells is not well understood; until about fifteen years ago, only three human diseases were attributable to *Bartonella* organisms.[1] We do know that patients infected with both *Borrelia* and *Bartonella* report abnormally high levels of neurological dysfunction. Some tick-borne illnesses have only been recently discovered. As such, some illnesses—like *Powassan encephalitis,* a virus that invades and infects the brain—have no known effective treatment options to date, and are potentially fatal.[2]

Any of these infections when paired with Lyme make the presentation of the disease significantly more complex and more difficult to diagnose. And yet, most patients diagnosed with Lyme disease are not tested for the other potential threats, generally because those tests are not widely available. For patients infected with all four major tick-borne illnesses, it's nearly impossible to avoid the effects of the advanced form of Lyme disease. This is the stage in which patients require the most assistance from doctors and loved ones, but many who reach late-stage Lyme find that support and assistance difficult to come by.

Both the Centers for Disease Control (CDC) and the Infectious Disease Society of America (IDSA) recommend two to six weeks of antibiotic treatment for patients whose blood tests confirm they're infected with Lyme disease. Both entities claim that after this treatment period patients are almost certainly cured of the infection—and thus they consider any additional antibiotic treatment superfluous. Much of the medical establishment claims it is impossible for spirochetes to survive in the body past this treatment, even if a patient has progressed into the final stages of infection. All the same, up to 20 percent of infected patients treated for Lyme disease do not get better.

The authors of the IDSA Lyme Treatment Guidelines label these persistent symptoms post-treatment Lyme syndrome, stating that, though they "sympathize with patients' suffering, [they] remain concerned that a diagnosis of so-called 'chronic Lyme disease,' suggesting that active infection is ongoing, is not supported by scientific evidence."[3] This statement, from 2012, is a significantly more sympathetic stance than the IDSA has taken previously. In its 2006 "Clinical Practice Guidelines" for Lyme disease, "Post-Treatment Lyme Syndrome" gets the following reference: "In many patients, post-treatment symptoms appear to be more related *to the aches and pains of daily living* [emphasis added] rather than to either Lyme disease or a tick-borne co-infection. Put simply, there is a relatively high frequency of the same kinds of symptoms in 'healthy' people."[4] Unfortunately, and despite the more compassionate phrasing in 2012, it's the 2006 document that's the worldwide standard for Lyme treatment, especially in countries where the infection is little known.

Yet even the more "sympathetic" 2012 statement speaks of "so-called 'chronic Lyme disease,'" a term that refers to continued presence of tick-borne infection and/or symptoms in a patient after the full prescribed course of antibiotic therapy. Some of these patients experience continued symptoms. Others "recover" from the infection and seem healthy again, only to experience sporadic "relapses" of Lyme symptoms; as such, some argue that these patients have never been completely cured of the disease.

Those who appear to be suffering from chronic Lyme often split into two subgroups. In the smaller group, encompassing perhaps less than half of sufferers, are the patients experiencing persistent symptoms who continue to test positive for the disease even after months or years of antibiotic treatment. In the much-larger group are patients who experience chronic symptoms without ever testing positive for the disease. Their diagnosis and treatment is based not on a blood test result, but on the litany of symptoms they experience and describe. These patients often find that antibiotics help manage their symptoms and keep their pain under control.

Arguably half the medical community doesn't believe such persistent symptoms are a physiological manifestation of Lyme infection. Instead, many believe the symptoms are psychological or psychosomatic, and choose not to treat. From the perspective of powerful institutions like the IDSA, the CDC, and the doctors who ally with them, it seems the argument for the existence of chronic Lyme disease is moot.

Despite these dismissive conclusions, many factors strengthen the argument for the existence of a "post-treatment Lyme syndrome." First is the inconsistent testing used to diagnose Lyme disease. Currently there are two primary tests used to diagnose Lyme: both seek out Lyme antibodies in the patients' blood, and are administered by a general practitioner, often getting negative results despite patient symptoms. The trouble is that both tests—the more common Enzyme-Linked Immunosorbent Assay (ELISA) and the Indirect Fluorescent Antibody (IFA) test—rely on technology developed during the 1980s. Many physicians estimate that these blood tests are accurate only 60 percent of the time. The other 40 percent of patients are sent home with false positive or false negative test results; some are never treated, even if they present a high number of Lyme symptoms.[5]

While most patients showing Lyme symptoms get one of the above two tests, a fair number of patients also receive the Polymerase Chain Reaction (PCR) Test, which scans the body for traces of spirochetal DNA. As this test is extremely expensive, it's often not employed. It's also extremely sensitive, to the extent it can produce positive results in patients *without* Lyme symptoms. Other patients receive spinal tap tests—but because spirochetes are to be found in spinal fluid during only some stages of a person's infection, this test can also be unreliable. The even-harder-to-come-by tests for other tick-borne co-infections are similarly inconsistent. Put simply, at this point there is no diagnostic test that can definitively determine whether or not a patient has been infected with Lyme disease—let alone how far along the infection has progressed. Despite the fact that it's widely known these tests are inconsistently reliable, some doctors, especially those outside the Lyme-predominant American Northeast, state that no patient should be treated for Lyme without scientific proof of infection. And so, many suffering from the disease are never treated for it, and many who continue to suffer past their treatment are denied additional treatment.

Unfortunately, it is the doctors who argue against the existence of chronic Lyme whose voices are heard the loudest, perhaps because they have the backing of major government health organizations and insurance companies. Fortunately, however, another group of doctors are speaking out as well, claiming Lyme should be recognized as potentially chronic and seriously damaging if symptoms continue after treatment. Many of these physicians claim that long-term antibiotic treatment, even IV treatment if necessary, helps to save their patients from debilitating disease.

Their evidence: they watch their patients get better. One doctor I spoke with "has no doubt about the existence of chronic Lyme." I asked her how she feels about the pushback she gets from conventional medicine about her stance on the illness. "I don't need someone to publish a study telling me chronic Lyme exists," she replied. "I see the proof walk in and out of my office every day."[6] If patients come in presenting Lyme symptoms, are treated with antibiotics, and then recover, she reasons, it seems to be a fair assumption that a bacterial infection was treated.

Respected scientific research does support these outlier diagnoses and practices. A recent Johns Hopkins study details a new method of testing for Lyme, exploring the ways *Borrelia* can persist in the body through cystic forms and in biofilm colonies, which, if present, wouldn't be identified by the standard tests for Lyme.[7] The standard round of antibiotics wouldn't treat these cysts and biofilm colonies; without that specific treatment, the patient will not be cured of the disease. But even encouraging studies such as these have their naysayers, as nearly every study suggesting the persistence of biological Lyme infection can be matched with another that denies it.

Though the medical establishment has reached no agreement, doctors on both sides of the debate approach their diagnoses with certainty. Most mainstream doctors base their diagnoses on test results; without a positive result, a patient receives no distinct diagnosis. Alternative physicians rely more on personal experience, and trust in patient descriptions. These are the doctors to whom Lyme patients flock when searching for treatment and answers.

These "Lyme-literate doctors" assert that chronic Lyme could be the result of spirochetes' resistance to antibiotics, a concept well-known to be a factor in the mutations of virulent bacteria and viruses.[8] Though the science is limited, there are a number of studies that have found spirochetes surviving in animal hosts after antibiotic treatment. One study, completed by the U.S. National Library of Medicine, demonstrated the persistence of spirochetal organisms in Rhesus monkeys even after long courses of both ceftriaxone and doxycycline.[9] Another study conducted by Columbia University Medical Center reached similar findings in mice.[10]

The post-treatment persistence of Lyme disease has been well documented in humans as well. In as early as 1993, active *Borrelia burgdorferi* was found in the spinal fluid of a patient who'd suffered with chronic septic Lyme arthritis of the knee for seven years—despite continuous antibiotic treatment.[11] That same year, a patient with Lyme-triggered blurred vision experienced persistent symptoms for several years after two separate month-long cycles of tetracycline. In this case, *Borrelia burgdorferi* was found in the patient's iris—proving the bacteria had moved beyond the blood stream.[12] And in 1994 the *New England Journal of Medicine* published a study on Lyme arthritis patients, which found the disease active and present in 37 percent of patients' spinal fluid after antibiotic therapy.[13] It's hard to understand how, despite the documentation of these cases and many more like them over twenty years ago, the medical establishment cannot agree that the disease can persist in the human body after a *single* course of antibiotics.

In seeking better understanding of Lyme disease, some doctors study the behavior of another spirochetal disease: syphilis. Dr. Nevena Zubcevik regards *Borrelia* as very similar to *Treponema*, the syphilis spirochete;[14] indeed, they share a subspecies, and their DNA are very similar. We now know that *Treponema* can lie dormant in animal hosts long after antibiotic treatment, and that times of high stress can trigger a relapse of the disease. And, like *Borrelia*, *Treponema* doesn't reside just in the blood; it can remain latent in other parts of the body as well. Today it's universally accepted that syphilis is both difficult to diagnose and treat and has the potential to persist after treatment—though universal agreement was not reached until the disease had been around for decades. The similarities are striking. Since majority opinion was originally wrong about the danger of syphilis, couldn't the same be true about a similar bacterium now? This isn't to say that Lyme disease behaves identically to syphilis; it does not. But their striking similarities certainly merit the consideration that additional scientific inquiry could in time demonstrate even greater similarity—which could only benefit all those suffering from either disease.

As it stands now, much remains to be understood. We know very little about the way spirochetes and other tick-borne viruses and bacteria interact within the human body, so it shouldn't be surprising that we know even less about the potential long-term effects of tick-borne illnesses. For one, recent research suggests Lyme disease can be transferred *in utero*, and can have lasting effects on fertility. In response to the September 2014 *Scientific American* article "Mothers May Pass Lyme Disease to Children in the Womb"[15] Dr. Richard Horowitz added to the conversation, stating that additional infections can also be transmitted to the fetus. "Other tick-borne infections, such as the relapsing fever spirochete, as well as *Babesia* and *Bartonella,* can also be transmitted to the fetus. Tick-borne infections represent a significant risk to pregnant women, and although the article states that there is little scientific evidence to suggest fetal malformations . . . , there are many scientific articles proving that Lyme can both harm and kill a developing fetus."[16] He went on to cite nineteen articles and studies. Note that this information is rarely shared with new patients of the disease.

A second angle concerns how in 2006 Dr. Alan MacDonald, an impassioned researcher who has studied Lyme disease for decades, presented alarming findings about a potential relationship between Lyme and Alzheimer's disease. In his study of ten Alzheimer patients, he found that the DNA of spirochetes had combined with human DNA in 70 percent of the brains he examined.[17]

Though studies on long-term effects are inconclusive, one statistic is very clear: rates of infection are disturbingly high. In the United States alone, 300,000 new cases of Lyme are reported to the Centers for Disease Control every year; the CDC also acknowledges that a large number of cases likely go unreported.[18] Given that, statistically, the standard antibiotic treatment will prove to be insufficient for 10 to 20 percent of new cases, that means 30,000 to 60,000 people each year will join the list of those dealing with chronic, persistent symptoms.

And while the U.S. debates around chronic Lyme make a debilitating illness even more strained, at least patients in the States have access to those debates. Australia, China, Japan, Singapore, and most European countries now also report high rates of infection— but most Lyme patients outside the U.S. receive the absolute minimum of information about their condition. Many doctors in Singapore, for example, have never heard of Lyme disease. In Australia, there are currently fifty doctors treating over 200,000 patients.[19]

As the rate of infection increases, the risk of infection seems to climb with it. The vast majority of cases are contracted in the Northeastern U.S., specifically in Dutchess County, New York, the most endemic county in the world. In an October 2014 article in the *Poughkeepsie Journal,* environmental scientist Taal Levi, who has studied environments from Brazil to Alaska, notes that, in terms of sheer numbers of infected ticks, no region scares him as much as Dutchess County. "The nature here is terrifying. It's more dangerous to walk around in the forest here than it is to walk around the forest in Brazil."[20] With no objective, agreed-upon understanding of how best to treat all Lyme patients, whose ranks grow every day, shouldn't this increased risk trigger extensive additional study, wherever the findings might lead us?

CHAPTER 3

OUR OWN BREED OF WARRIOR

It was spring of 2006. I was sitting in a circle with six other fifteen-year-old girls and a bottle of vodka playing Truth or Dare. The rules of the game dictated that if someone didn't want to complete a dare or answer a question, they took a drink. Simple. Apparently safe.

We started with easy truth questions. What color underwear are you wearing? What's your favorite food? How old were you the first time you kissed a boy? I took the first drink when asked about my morning routine. The other girls were surprised I chose not to reveal what I did each morning. I didn't want to share how I had to talk myself through standing up and putting on my clothes every morning, that when I pulled up my jeans it felt like my skin was falling off. I didn't reveal how zipping and buttoning the top of my pants seemed impossible when my hands felt like they were on fire. I couldn't say it out loud because I was scared they wouldn't believe me, because I was scared I wouldn't believe the words coming out of my own mouth. So instead I smiled and drank, and pretended I lived in someone else's body.

In the town where I grew up, everyone knew about Lyme. "Easy to diagnose and simple to treat," people said. "As long as you get the medicine in you, you'll be fine." So many people had been diagnosed in our neighborhood that most fancied themselves Lyme experts. But the Lyme disease everyone talked about was not the Lyme disease my father knew, or the one I would eventually come to know.

I wondered sometimes if my dad also kept his experience secret from his friends, hiding behind the preconceived notions that Lyme is as easily conquered as a bad sinus infection. I'm embarrassed that I can't easily recall images of him during the peaks of his illness. I do have one memory of him: sitting limp in the large armchair in our living room. His face was gray, his eyes glossed over, the energy drained from his body. Though my father had been sick with Lyme from the time of my own infection, I never associated the illness with him. To me the PICC line (peripherally inserted central catheter, part of his antibiotic treatment) in his arm was more like Inspector Gadget than illness, and when he stopped working, I understood nothing more than that he spent more time reading to us before bed. I didn't notice the hardship my dad experienced; I never saw a rash or a cut. To me, his Lyme disease was invisible.

Even at his sickest we spent our winter weekends in Vermont, driving every Friday night to ski the following morning. My dad self-administered IV antibiotics en route, one hand on the wheel, the other lying still on the center consol. I don't know how this didn't scare or worry me, but I was convinced he was stronger than ever. During some of our weekly drives I fought my heavy eyelids, wanting to stay awake with him through the night. Resting my head against the humming window, I'd watch his fingers effortlessly drumming along to U2, his smiling eyes focused intently on the road.

The day drives we spent playing. All seven of us spent hours singing show tunes at the top of our lungs or looking for letters of the alphabet along the highway.

"If a fern tree and a pine tree had a baby, what kind of tree would it be?" I once asked.

"Ummm, Oak?" my mom replied.

"Maple?" Meg called out.

"Nope and nope."

"It would be a *Fine* tree," my dad screamed.

"Correct! The winner is Dad Cashel!!!" Everyone cheered while I came up with the next question and its pre-determined next winner.

I remember my dad's hands moved from the blinker back to the wheel with instinctual ease, and when he looked into the rear view mirror he simultaneously smiled at me, called out an answer, and checked the lane behind him.

On one of our nighttime drives, I asked if he had to split his eyes in order to look at the road and me at the same time.

"No," he answered. "It's a road warrior skill. Both your eyes are always engaged when you're out on the highway. You'll understand one day."

He always called himself that: road warrior. On the road, he was free— or at least he had the potential to be. I wonder sometimes if he felt as free as I imagined. Did pain and stiffness test his agile turns of the steering wheel? Did his veins burn as the medicine pumped through them?

No one in my family was very much in touch with his illness. He worked to keep it private, and we never resisted that effort. Knowing what I do now, I wish I could go back and hug him more gently, or let him go to sleep instead of demanding he keep reading. Someone once told me they had never felt empathy until they experienced intense physical pain. I wonder sometimes if I am the same way.

While my dad was sick, my world was cozily small. Nothing was bigger than home. And however busy each day might be, with rehearsals or classes after school, each night I came home again to the safety and routine of our family kitchen. There may have been television news running in the background, or Mom might have been talking on the phone, her attention somewhere far away, but all that resonated with me was the food cooking on the stove, the quiet privacy of our kitchen.

Our home held another thing I kept private: a discomfort I thought was normal. Each day, my knees and fingers swelled, and almost every time I took a step, or lifted a pencil, the added pressure in my joints made me feel like they were grinding against each other, working too hard against an unwelcome resistance. By middle school my heart could start racing for no reason, and five minutes could pass without my realizing it. Though these sound serious now, at the time I easily rationalized away my symptoms as the growing pains of adolescence.

With age my world started to grow. And as I spent time with more kids my age I started to sense my body experienced something much different from theirs. The realization that my discomforts were definitively abnormal came on the morning of my eighth-grade graduation as I waited my turn to receive my diploma. I felt a film of sweat cover me like another layer of skin, starting at the back of my neck and spreading slowly up my skull, down my spine, out to my limbs, until I felt I could no longer breathe. Focused on keeping up appearances, I fought to keep my eyes open, to keep my feet supporting my body as I followed the procession. With every step fluid expanded in my joints until they felt ready to burst. After I received my diploma, I could think only of where the nearest place was to sit down. It was exhausting.

Afterward, a Lyme specialist who'd been in the audience approached my parents and said, "I think your daughter is very, very sick. She needs to come see me."

At first, my second diagnosis with Lyme disease seemed like a new infection. It wasn't until later conversations that I linked my symptoms over the previous years to a resurgence of my original infection. My doctor recommended a new treatment plan, this time delivered intravenously in the hopes that a concentrated treatment would permanently annihilate the spirochetes still plaguing me. We knew very little of the mainstream medical opinions about Lyme disease at the time, and any concern about the speed with which I was diagnosed or the aggressive nature of treatment was trumped by the realization that something had been so wrong, for so long. I was ashamed of my ignorance; not only of my own situation, but also of the way it had mirrored my father's, something we all had chosen not to see.

I know it's strange that I spent years developing symptoms of a disease my father had also experienced, yet we never acknowledged the pattern. So much of my dad's experience with Lyme was kept private, secret even. I wasn't familiar with the sensations of his disease, and thus was unable to recognize them in myself. We didn't have a shared language or vocabulary that we could use to talk about it, so until someone re-introduced us to it, our denial prevented us from finding the connection between our two experiences.

I started IV treatment that summer, and continued receiving IV Rocephin every morning once school started, with a larger dose on the weekends. I saved my higher dose for days that I didn't have school because my body tended to react negatively if the drug was administered for more than a half hour. I always felt burning in my arms during treatment, but on longer drips my veins would often collapse, and I would need to have my needle reinserted, a process I could only tolerate once each day before school.

The clinic was in the windowless basement of my doctor's home. Though she had refurbished it to look like a standard doctor's office, the space was tired. The wallpaper peeled near the ceiling, revealing concrete walls. Mismatched chairs lined these walls: some standard waiting room seats, others possibly pulled from the kitchen table upstairs. Every morning my nurse waddled into the treatment room, greeting returning patients as she wheeled my medication behind her. When she tapped her long fingernails against the metal IV stand, I couldn't help but notice the warts on her fingers and hands. She did not wear gloves. "Don't worry sweetheart," she'd say, the corners of her lips framed by white chunks of saliva, "I'm very good at my job." Then she'd kneel beside me. "You ready, baby?" I always lied. She'd then prepare the needle, put the tourniquet on my arm, and tell me to close my eyes. We did this together every day for six months.

Three months in, when I started high school in September, my track marks seemed more noticeable, my IV trips more frustrating. As the veins in my arms became less accessible, we often had to resort to my wrists and hands, where the bruising was more apparent. All the patients with whom I had started treatment had now finished their course, so I became the dreary, senior patient—no longer part of the new crop of wide-eyed patients coming in.

Still, I never endured a drip on my own. My mom sat with me almost every morning, and arranged for a surrogate to sit with me on the rare days she missed. When school was cancelled one snow day, my drip turned into a breakfast date: we stopped to pick up muffins and sodas at the café on the way, a treat my siblings were never to hear about. Afterward we headed to the nearly empty nail salon for semi-private manicures.

But, despite Mom's efforts to make the treatment bearable, by December my patience was wearing as thin as my veins. She took her support to a new level. After telling me she'd been feeling tired and achy, she asked my doctor to treat her for Lyme as well. Our doctor put my mother on IV Rocephin without testing her, and without a proper symptom diagnosis. For the last month of my treatment, my mother didn't sit with me every day in support, but now also for her own IV drip.

This gave me a new reason to be there, and an opportunity to focus on supporting her rather than on my own experience. But, as much as I treasure her immensely loving gesture, her attempt to normalize my condition—emphasizing I wasn't deranged, I wasn't abnormal—I also knew there was something very wrong with our doctor.

As a result, I started to doubt my own experience of Lyme disease.

If my doctor would treat someone who wasn't sick, maybe I wasn't sick either. Maybe my pain was in my head, and my treatment had more to do with a crazy doctor who filled her office with kitchen chairs than with my own condition. Still, my pain and sensitivity had improved, my headaches were less frequent, and I felt healthy for the first time in over a year. Mom came to the clinic for about two months, after which we both stopped treatment. I decided I was okay. How couldn't I be?

As winter turned to spring, I worked hard to build myself up mentally. This included convincing myself I was cured despite the fact that I felt myself degenerating. I lost weight, but my face, my eyes, even my nose felt swollen. I was drowning internally.

In March of 2006, my parents called Dr. Bernard Raxlen to arrange my first official consult since my tests in 1998. In working with the last doctor we had hoped we were pursuing treatment we wouldn't have gotten from Dr. Raxlen; it felt like a step backward to return to him now.

We sat with him for more than two hours charting my symptoms over the last eight years. I tested positive for Lyme as well as for three other blood diseases, *Ehrlichiosis, Bartonella*, and *Babesia*. This was the first time I'd heard the words *Bartonella* and *Babesia*, the two untreated co-infections that caused some of my most debilitating symptoms. It became clear to me during that visit that I had to stop desperately trying to keep my identity separate from illness. If I wanted to get better, I had to name and understand what was happening in my body.

After an initial treatment of oral antibiotics and supplements produced little improvement, Dr. Raxlen recommended twice-daily antibiotics administered intravenously via a PICC line: a catheter to my heart. I wasn't scared. I had watched my father do it lots of times, and it looked easier than the endless early morning trips to get my daily IV. I saw this new method as a convenience—one that meant I could get my treatment at home, immersed in a book or in front of the TV without needles or pain.

I remember the white shirt I wore that day, with sleeves short enough to permit insertion of the plastic vein. Before we left I took a picture of my arm in the mirror, just in case I forgot what it looked like without a catheter.

When we arrived at Dr. Raxlen's waiting room I sat again on his leather couch and greeted the teddy bear across the room as my seven-year-old self had done nine years earlier. The armchair that once held the sick woman was empty, and I found myself missing her presence. Though I hadn't been carried in, I was now the sickest patient, once again the veteran in the room. When we entered the treatment room we were greeted by the same chatty nurse who'd inserted my father's catheter years before.

A peripherally inserted central catheter, which gets threaded through a vein up toward the heart, enables intravenous antibiotics to be directly pumped throughout the patient's body. Proper insertion requires that the patient be awake and aware as a large pencil-sized needle is inserted into the arm. I lay on my back, my left arm laid out straight as if strapped to the table, my head faced away from my parents. The nurse made a joke as he wiped the sweat off of my forehead, telling me it was going to be okay. I heard my mom take a deep breath, and then I felt the needle.

Aching is not the right word. *Stabbing* is not the right word. Not even *sharp*. I felt open. I felt like I could feel the nurse's breath penetrating the pencil-thick hole in my arm. My eyes focused on a crack in the wall, my thoughts wandering to death from oxygen injection. If I was open, if my veins were open, couldn't the air kill me? The room was silent. And then I felt my new vein.

Before my youngest brother learned to crawl he dragged himself along the wood floor. His belly never separating from the ground, building resistance. That's what the tube felt like as it moved through my arm: resistance. My body begged it to move with less friction, less pain. The crack in the wall was growing. As the vein made its way toward my heart I had to turn my head farther to the right, closer to the swelling crack, to ease its passage. Once it passed the bend of my shoulder I couldn't feel it anymore; I felt nothing when it pinched the outside of my heart.

There was blood, the sleeve of my white shirt stained red. But soon everything was clean: I changed my shirt, I was eating a cookie, conversation started up again as they showed us how to pump the medicine into my chest. I remember laughing, and how when I saw the sadness behind my parents' smiles I thought I would throw up.

Nurses were supposed to visit our house weekly to clean the PICC line and change my dressing, but I wouldn't let anyone other than my father touch it. He was the only person who knew how it felt to be so open: so violated, threatened by oxygen. He was the only person who would clean the line gently, who would cover what I didn't want to see with white, pristine gauze and clean tape. His movements were so precise and calculated that he'd sweat through his clothes during each dressing change. I always knew he would do it right.

The only time my dad and I had a PICC line mishap was one week before it was to be removed. While trying to cut some gauze away he accidentally snipped part of the line resting on my arm. I felt nothing, but I could see pain and fear tear through him. As the color drained from his face blood dripped out of the new hole in my tube. When I saw the blood I felt only relief, knowing it would have to be removed, that I wouldn't have to carry it around like a flag announcing I was sick.

We went to the emergency room to get the line removed, and before receiving any treatment endured criticism from the technicians about my father's handling procedures only a certified nurse should do. I didn't realize then that every medical appointment added a page to my file—and that, as my file got thicker and thicker, so grew an equal prejudice against me. The longer I stayed sick, the lower were my chances my case would be treated fairly and objectively.

I once thought I was lucky to have been diagnosed with Lyme rather than another disease. I now realize it wasn't Lyme that had made my experience relatively manageable—it was the people around me. Few other Lyme patients receive the incredible level of support I had during the first eight years of my experience. Starting with year nine, I became intimately familiar with the more negative experiences shared by Lyme patients around the world—when I lost faith in my own perceptions in the hands of the medical personnel supposedly caring for me.

CHAPTER 4

THE BIAS AGAINST CHRONIC LYME

The debate over the existence of chronic Lyme disease adds a layer of hardship to what is already a painful, confusing experience—the psychological effect of living with a disease many do not speak of, and that some don't even believe in, can at times equal its physical weight. Much of this debate concerns the lack of ongoing research, which limits both the quality and quantity of information available to doctors and patients. Essentially, opponents of chronic Lyme reason that there is not much need to research further what we already know: that the bacterium cannot survive the standard treatment. Even though the Lyme-causing bacterium was first identified in 1981, it wasn't until 2006 that the CDC updated their treatment guidelines to include prophylactic—"preventative" antibiotic— treatment for patients displaying a bull's-eye rash, even without a positive blood test.[21] The pace of Lyme's research history is much more sluggish than that of otherwise similar infections. Though it's true that governmental processing is notoriously slow in all arenas, there does appear to be another censoring force at work, one that both inhibits study and discourages open discussion.

In preparation for a June 2012 special on Lyme disease, the producers of WBUR, Boston's NPR news station, sought out many doctors to speak on the topic. In the end only three agreed to speak, two of them only anonymously; many other doctors never returned repeated phone calls. One doctor who declined cited the environment as "simply to volatile" for him to state his opinion. Kathleen McNerney, the producer of *Morning Edition*, told CommonHealth.WBUR.org she "could not think of a another medical field where it is more difficult to find a doctor to speak on the record."[22]

Doctors who ally themselves with the chronic Lyme population fear media appearances because such can make them targets of both medical disciplinary review boards and the insurance industry. Insurance companies work strenuously to revoke the medical licenses of doctors reputed as treating chronic Lyme—"Lyme-literate doctors," often called LLMDs—by asking their patients to file malpractice suits against them.[23] In another approach, insurance companies scour medical records for small inconsistencies in note-taking or record-keeping, bringing doctors to court on charges apparently separate from their Lyme treatments.[24] And of course the insurance companies regularly drop patients whose treatment exceeds the IDSA recommendations.[25]

Fortunately, New York State recently passed S7854, the "physician protection bill," which "prohibits the investigation of any claim" of medical misconduct "based solely on treatment that is not universally accepted by the medical profession": essentially, the bill protects New York doctors who treat Lyme disease after the recommended four-week treatment. Because the IDSA and CDC do not support the belief that Lyme can persist in the body post treatment, those opposed objected to the government intervening on behalf of doctors prescribing unproven treatments for an unproven disease. Similar laws have already been passed in New Hampshire, Connecticut, Rhode Island, and Maine. Following suit on the national level, in September 2014 the House of Representatives passed the Tick-Borne Disease Research Transparency and Accountability Act, "bipartisan legislation which prioritizes federal research on Lyme and related diseases and gives patients, advocates, and physicians a seat at the table." This was both the first stand-alone bill addressing Lyme disease to make it through the House and the first to create a safe space for all perspectives to be heard.[26]

To understand what a long time coming that safe space has been, consider the saga of New York doctor Richard Horowitz. In the early 1990s, Dr. Horowitz started noticing symptoms of *Babesia* in his patients. When blood samples came back positive, he informed the New York State health department, stating he believed a new disease in the blood supply needed to be addressed. The health department reported they believed the blood tests to be incorrect. Undaunted, Horowitz then tested a collection of ticks in the area for *Babesia,* sending the subsequent positive results to the governor. He was again told the test results had to be wrong—and was quickly removed from two organizations via which members can conduct tests in nationally recognized labs.[27] He has since gone on to treat patients of Lyme, *Babesia*, and other tick-borne illnesses with great success at the Healing Arts Center in Hyde Park, New York. His recent book on tick-borne illness—or what he calls "multiple systemic infectious disease syndrome"—*Why Can't I Get Better?: Solving the Mystery of Lyme and Chronic Disease,* is now a *New York Times* best seller. Yet this is a doctor who was, and to some extent still is, deemed a "quack" by many in the mainstream medical field.

While the hope of legal protection will aid many LLMDs and their patients, we still have much ground to cover. Since the original U.S. outbreak in the 1970s, doctors and scientists have struggled to publish in mainstream medical journals studies supporting the existence of *chronic* Lyme.[28] In stark contrast, in 1999, Dr. Gary Wormser, one of the doctors who helped author the CDC and IDSA guidelines, found quick publication of his discovery of *Babesia* in a placenta, despite the fact that this came years after Dr. Horowitz attempted to alert the health department of its presence in the blood supply.[29] Why are some scientists and their findings supported and others not? Why is research on chronic Lyme denied equal attention? Isn't it the role of science to continue asking questions?

It isn't just the medical journals that have been stunningly biased against chronic Lyme: mainstream media also favors the CDC and IDSA minimalist parameters on the disease. For example, a 2012 *New York Times* article entitled "Re-Infection not Relapses Brings Back Lyme Symptoms," claimed that scientists had proven chronic Lyme could not persist past antibiotic treatment in the body: that any patients presenting symptoms after treatment had to have been reinfected, that they had not experienced "relapses" of the original infection.[30] The article cites the reappearance of the bull's eye rash as proof of reinfection, but offers no explanation for patients who continue to display symptoms without a new bite or rash. This rather old information is presented as new "proof" debunking chronic Lyme.

We can cite some progress. On July 1, 2013, the *New Yorker* published Michael Specter's "The Lyme Wars," which presented a more balanced view of both the medical and political landscape and the experience of patients living with chronic Lyme. The article particularly highlights the lack of information and research about the disease, as well as the debate over the validity of chronic Lyme.[31] This is not to say that Specter stands firmly in the chronic Lyme camp. During an NPR interview he revealed that, even after interviewing and speaking to numerous patients of chronic Lyme, he still didn't believe those with negative test results were suffering from an actual infection. (Note that Specter is a journalist by trade, not a physician.) He continued by saying the development of diagnostic tests should be the priority for researchers and doctors right now.[32] As much as the chronic Lyme proponents dislike the institutional stance based solely on test results, there would be benefit to both sides were we to develop comprehensive tests that reliably detected the bacterium wherever it hides in the body.

That said, patients suffering from Lyme cannot wait for the next diagnostic breakthrough, and still have to contend with doctors who don't understand what they experience. For now, the best we can hope for is to find medical practitioners who trust that the symptoms we describe are physiological rather than psychological—that they're not just in our heads.

Fortunately for Lyme patients, as time passes more about chronic Lyme is seeing print. As of about 2013 mainstream media is finally speaking about Lyme disease with more regularity, focusing on the high number of undiagnosed or misdiagnosed patients, or on the rising number of individuals infected in the United States each year. Unfortunately, though a notable percentage of these patients will join those experiencing chronic symptoms, and this more contentious post-treatment issue remains relatively untouched by the media.[33]

This is not the case for the *Poughkeepsie Journal*, which lies in the heart of Dutchess County, New York, one of the most Lyme-endemic areas in the world. The *Poughkeepsie Journal* often publishes articles by journalists such as Jill Auerbach, who has been a vital resource for those interested in staying abreast of Lyme politics and research. But, for those outside the Lyme community, information and publication about this disease is shockingly rare, despite the growing number of those newly infected each year.

The lack of dialogue about chronic Lyme perpetuates the belief that Lyme disease does not pose a significant risk to the population. And because so few write or speak about the disease, patients are often disinclined to speak about it themselves. As such, the conversation ends before it begins.

A few theories may explain some of the intention behind this pervasive bias. One is told by Michael Christopher Carroll in his book *Lab 257: The Disturbing Story of the Government's Secret Plum Island Germ Laboratory*. On Plum Island, a small island just two miles the coast of Old

Lyme, Connecticut, Lab 101 and Lab 257 were established for animal disease research after World War II with the intention of protecting America against threats of biological warfare from the Soviet Union. The labs were designed and run by two men: William Arthur Hagan, a veterinarian and former dean of Cornell University's veterinary school; and Erich Traub, a Nazi germ warfare expert who had worked for Heinrich Himmler, after which he was smuggled into the States to work for the CIA and the U. S. Department of Agriculture, forgiven of all war crimes. Strange bedfellows to be sure.

In painting a detailed picture of the inner workings of lab 257, Carroll makes two alarming claims: both labs hold many of the most dangerous species of bacteria in the world, and both are dangerously unprotected. He connects the open-air testing done in the labs with the appearance of diseases like Lyme, West Nile virus, and Dutch Duck plague, all of which made their first U.S. appearance only a few miles from Plum Island. Similarly, the Lone Star Tick, previously found in only certain parts of Texas, emerged on the East Coast as well. All of these presented *after* the labs were established. Carroll's claim that the U.S. government has a vested interest in blocking research on Lyme disease—out of concern for maintaining the confidentiality of Plum Island[34]—is a tantalizing one that, if true, would explain a great deal.

I do want to note that with the exception of Carroll's book, most descriptions of the classified relationship between Plum Island and Lyme disease tend to be biased and hyperbolic—reading most likely to be found in grocery store checkout lines. All the same, the Department of Homeland Security's own statements about the research conducted there should not be taken lightly. As of October 2013, the Science and Technology section of the DHS website stated that "the Plum Island Animal Disease Center is a Biosafety Level 3 (BSL-3) facility designed and constructed to work with the most dangerous animal diseases in the world, such as foot-and-mouth disease (FMD), Rinderpest, and African swine fever. In fact, by federal law, Plum Island is the only place in the U.S. where FMD and Rinderpest viruses can be studied."[35] The site additionally confirms that, though experiments in bio warfare have been conducted on the island, biological weapons developed there are not meant for use against humans. They instead target the human food supply—hence the classification as an animal disease lab.

Of particular interest to me is how this lab classifies the disease. Do the researchers at Plum Island believe Lyme disease has the potential to be a weapon of biological warfare? As it turns out, they do. In 2010, a journalist from the ASX Digital Group asked a similar question, after which she discovered that, at the opening of the Margaret Batts Tobin Laboratory Building in Texas, the CDC stated the facility would be used to study such diseases as anthrax, tularemia, cholera, Lyme disease, desert valley fever, and other parasitic and fungal diseases. The Centers for Disease Control and Prevention identified these diseases as "potential bioterrorism agents."[36]

Let's return to undeniable facts we have about Plum Island. We know that the researchers on Plum Island conducted open-air testing on ticks. We know there was research and experiments conducted in bio warfare. If the CDC today includes Lyme in its list of potential bioterrorism agents, isn't it possible, even likely, that the researchers on Plum Island saw Lyme similarly? We can not definitively say that Lyme disease originated on Plum Island, or that our government was responsible for the original outbreak. But we can ask: why is the government spending time and money studying the "bioterrorism" potential of a disease they also claim can be cured with a standard treatment of antibiotics lasting at most six weeks?

Regardless of the various ramifications of this subject, it does seem as though the United States, specifically the CDC, is well aware of the power of *Borrelia burgdorferi*, a force sufferers of chronic Lyme disease know all too well. So why have the CDC and most of the mainstream medical community not yet admitted the same?

Perhaps, as stated earlier, the government simply wants to keep secret its dangerous treatment of some of the world's most deadly species of bacteria. But there are other possible theories for the code of silence around chronic Lyme. One of the most common posits that insurance companies have a vested financial interest in keeping the approved treatment as short as possible. This strikes me as a viable theory—with at least two puzzling exceptions.

The first concerns the fact that doxycycline, the tetracycline antibiotic used to treat a number of bacterial infections, including Lyme, is prescribed by doctors and approved by insurance companies for years at a time for a more benign purpose: to treat acne. This is curious, given that CDC and IDSA cite fear of doing harm as their rationale for denying Lyme patients longer-term antibiotic treatment, stating: "Using antibiotics for a very long time (months or years) does not offer superior results and in fact can be dangerous, because it can cause potentially fatal complications."[37] If this is the case, then why do acne patients receive continued antibiotic treatment?

To further this inquiry, let's look at the doses for each purpose. According to Johns Hopkins Medicine, Lyme patients are usually prescribed 100 mg doxycycline, taken orally twice daily for three to six weeks.[38] Compare this to the standard prescription for acne: 100 mg orally, taken twice a day for three to six weeks or until improvement occurs; followed by a maintenance dose of 50 to 150 mg orally once a day.[39]

Doxycycline is also approved by the CDC to prevent malaria; their "Medicines for the Prevention of Malaria While Traveling" states: "CDC has no limits on the use of doxycycline for the prevention of malaria. There is no evidence of harm when the drug has been used for extended periods of time." Note that the dosage for malaria prevention is the same as that for acne and Lyme.[40]

Returning to the theory that the code of silence around chronic Lyme might derive from insurance companies' vested interest in limiting treatment: the second puzzling exception is that Lyme disease costs the health care system an exorbitant, and perhaps unnecessary, amount of money. New research out of Johns Hopkins Bloomberg School of Public Health suggests Lyme disease "costs the U.S. healthcare system between $712 million and $1.3 billion a year—or nearly $3,000 per patient on average—in return doctor visits and testing, likely to investigate the cause of some patients' lingering symptoms of fatigue, musculoskeletal pain, and memory problems. These visits come after patients have finished their original course of antibiotics." According to these researchers, patients with Lyme have nearly "87 percent more visits to the doctor and 71 percent more visits to the emergency room within the year following [their] diagnosis. Those with Lyme disease were nearly 5 times more likely to have any [post-treatment Lyme disease syndrome]-related diagnosis—fatigue, nerve pain, joint pain, cognitive troubles—within that year and were 5.5 times more likely to have a diagnosis of debility and excessive fatigue."[41] If these patients were treated more aggressively and successfully from the start, wouldn't these costs be significantly lower?

I don't know why there exists such a bias against the existence of chronic Lyme; experts in the field have not reached a unanimous conclusion, and I can't seem to find a satisfying one myself. While I won't name names, I can share information I received from several Lyme-literate doctors. In requesting their thoughts on the pushback regarding research, testing, treatment, and general awareness of chronic Lyme disease, I was told by two doctors they simply did not know. Another believes the U.S. government doesn't want to admit there is an infectious disease epidemic on American soil. Yet another doctor is sure Carroll had it right. One considers the pushback entirely financially driven. And another doctor stated with great confidence it's because people don't want to hear about Lyme—

that they're scared of it. "Denial is a powerful thing," he said, "I think that's what the problem is. No one wants to talk about it. Healthy people talk to healthy people. Lyme patients talk to other Lyme patients. Doctors talk to other doctors. There isn't any crossover, [so] no one gets to understand the other side of the debate."

CHAPTER 5

FACT BECOMES FICTION

Just before I started my senior year of high school in September 2008, my dad took me to see Dr. Raxlen to try to understand the nerve-racking symptoms I'd started displaying that summer. Dr. Raxlen was the doctor who had diagnosed my Lyme disease ten years earlier, whose office I had visited many times since. Though my recent symptoms were unlike any I'd had in the past, Dr. Raxlen had watched me fall in and out of illness for years, so he'd have insight few other physicians would. I remember sitting in his office with my father, who at his sickest dealt with very similar neurological problems to the ones I was experiencing that summer. I sat on the examination table wringing my hands, pinching the insides of my palms to try to stay focused and present through our conversation. My vision was spotty, and the sound of Dr. Raxlen's voice swelled and dissolved with the dynamics of a large orchestra.

"I would encourage you to get a second opinion," he said to my dad, watching me out of the corner of his eye, "but be careful not to rule out Lyme here. It's not unheard of for patients to experience the emergence of new symptoms, especially during times of high pressure or stress." I don't remember what we said back to him, or how we got home after the appointment. I do remember being scared, confused, and frustrated by the foreign nature of my brain. It did not seem like Lyme disease to me, but then again, I had never experienced the neurological side of Lyme before.

The following month of my life is basically lost to my memory—about some days and weeks I know only what I've been told. I know that in the first week of school I auditioned for my senior play, *The Rimers of El-dritch,* and that afterward I called my mom to talk about it. After I hung up the phone, I called her again, initiating the same conversation. The next morning at school I apologized to my English teacher for not doing my homework; she told me I'd emailed it to her the night before. A few days later I came downstairs from my bedroom and did not recognize Heather or the house I had lived in since I was ten years old. I do remember a read-through for the play I was cast in—I got the part of Mary Windrod. When I looked at my script, I was unable to make out the meanings of the sentences. Some single words were recognizable, but others became meaningless lines of symbols I couldn't begin to pronounce. The next day I dropped out of the play, resigned that I couldn't manage the role. Soon after, my parents decided I needed to join them in Massachusetts.

In the third week of September, Heather and Calvin drove me to my parents' house in Hingham, Massachusetts. I couldn't sit up on the drive. For days I hadn't been able to eat much more than yogurt. Music made me feel I was going to throw up, and the headlights tore through my eyes and pierced my brain. I lay in the backseat on Calvin's lap as he rubbed my back. All the while, Heather, still a relative stranger, patiently pushed the car forward through the rain.

For the first few weeks back with my parents I slept about eighteen hours a day. Words had become almost entirely foreign to me. I couldn't read or write, and had developed a frustrating stammer that made the conversation I craved nearly impossible. I was extremely sensitive to light and sound, and was in constant pain: muscle pain, joint pain, head pain. At times, it was inescapable.

On some days I couldn't leave my room, but there were days when I had slightly more energy. I'd take advantage of the small amounts time when I felt more like myself to talk to Calvin on the phone, or watch my mom practice yoga in the living room. Small things, like going for a ride in the car, felt like big victories then. It's hard for me to describe now, but I remember that I had to live from moment to moment. When I felt okay, I tried to fully embrace those minutes of feeling okay; when I was in pain, I would have wait for that pain to pass. I didn't have the energy to think further ahead than the next hour or the next day, but if by some stroke of luck I had a better hour than the last, it didn't go unnoticed.

Moving just outside of Boston had been a stroke of luck: Boston was the epicenter of America's mainstream medical system, and Boston's doctors were among the best educated in the country. If they couldn't help me, perhaps no one could. Thanks to a close friend of my aunt, I was able to get appointment with the head of the pediatrics department at one of the major hospitals in the city. He would oversee a diagnosis and treatment plan across a multitude of disciplines—"the best doctors in the world," they crowed; they would put "100 percent" effort into my case—whatever was needed to get me back on my feet. The enthusiasm and dedication I was promised before they saw my medical history was inspiring, even exciting.

I was having a good morning the day of my initial visit. I remember my mom and I laughed for most of the drive to the hospital. We laughed at the funny GPS voice and at Boston's disorganized streets, so different from the familiar grid back in New York. I remember the energy between us was refreshing and light.

It was a forty-five-minute wait in yet another waiting room before my new doctor, an adolescent psychiatrist, came out to greet us for our sole in-person meeting. He shook my hand too hard, squeezing it tight. When he let go, the blood rushed into my hand, and I knew he wasn't going to help me.

He then took my mother into his office, leaving me alone in the waiting room. He asked my mom about my medical history, about my thoughts on my illness. He asked my mom to describe how I had felt during all I'd endured. For two hours I waited for someone to treat *me*, not my medical file, not others' interpretations of my experience. When they came back out two hours later, my mom didn't make eye contact with me. He said goodbye, and we left.

My mother cried on the drive home. Her energy is always so alive, so imaginative, so focused and passionate, but then she was deflated. The doctor had peremptorily dismissed her first mention of Lyme, citing it an impossibility. He'd told her my present symptoms most likely were a display representing the abandonment I felt about my family's move. He'd told her I was regressing, and had chastised her about the aggressive Lyme treatment I'd received, criticizing her trust in the doctors we had chosen. At one point he'd even asked: "During all these years, did it not occur to you to take this child to a children's hospital?," thus shattering her trust in our experience of the past four years. Without spending even one minute with me, this medical hero had determined I suffered from a psychological breakdown, not an infectious disease—a diagnosis likely reached before he even came out to greet us. This didn't mean he wasn't going to oversee my treatment; he was—but he had quickly dismissed Lyme as the source of my suffering.

In an effort to "check all the boxes," he did refer me to an infectious disease pediatrician later that week—and this time my dad joined us as well. This doctor was a nicer man. He took the time to examine my body, and learned firsthand how much pain I felt in certain areas, and how little sensation I felt in others. He heard me struggle to speak, saw how my eyes darted away from the sharp pain of light. After his examination he told us that, while my symptoms were very similar to those of untreated, late-stage Lyme disease, it was nearly impossible I actually had Lyme. Spirochetes could not survive past a few months of antibiotic treatment, he told us, so there was no way they were still present after multiple years. As he spoke, the muscles in my legs shook uncontrollably.

"Is that true for every patient?" my father inquired.

"Studies suggest that it is the case for nearly 90 percent of patients infected with the disease."

"What about the other 10 percent?"

The doctor told us that, though he didn't know, that unknown 10 percent of patients didn't affect his diagnosis. Yes, those patients continued to show post-treatment symptoms of Lyme, but to him those symptoms were not the product of biological infection. He then asked my dad to compare the bank where he worked, a conservative, mainstream institution.

"That's what this hospital is too, Michael," he said with pride. "We're a conservative, right-down-the-middle-of-the-road kind of hospital. The IDSA says to treat Lyme disease for six weeks with antibiotics, and that is what we do. If the antibiotics don't work, then we aren't dealing with Lyme. That is what they say, so that is what we say."

"But what about the other 10 percent of people who still show symptoms after that six weeks?" Though my dad pressed, the doctor couldn't give him a good answer. "If the drugs make her feel better, and they won't kill her, can we at least give them a try?"

Simple and safe guidelines dictate the Lyme diagnosis process; the patients themselves are almost unnecessary. What is the benefit of this medical depersonalization? It safeguards doctors' accountability. After all, they can't get into trouble if they never take risks. So then why are these Boston physicians considered "leading" doctors when they follow rather than lead?

There are a number of true risks associated with long-term antibiotic therapy, concerns that dictate the decisions of doctors like the pediatrician I visited. To follow are just two of those risks. The first: since antibiotics kill all bacteria, even the microorganisms that help us stay healthy, patients who undergo long-term antibiotic therapy can struggle to maintain normal flora levels, which promote healthy digestion. The second and perhaps most threatening side effect of long-term antibiotic use is increased resistance to antibiotic therapy, whereby some bacteria are unaffected by the antibiotic, and can grow unabated. As a result, drugs developed to help us today may not be as effective tomorrow. We can develop antibiotic resistance when antibiotics are provided unnecessarily.

That said, if a patient is suffering from an infection, antibiotics can be necessary, even lifesaving. So, in the doctor's office that time—actually, anytime I consulted a doctor—we circled back to the basic question of whether or not I suffered from an infection. Either a bacterium was causing my illness, or it was not. If infection was indeed the cause of my illness, the benefits of prolonged antibiotic use outweighed the risks. But if it was not the cause, antibiotic therapy was not worth the risk.

To his credit, albeit his reluctance, the pediatrician prescribed a brief course of penicillin in the "highly unlikely" event that some bacterium was causing my pain. He also took blood tests and referred me to a psychiatrist, who he was sure would help much more than the medicine. From there we continued the medical maze into November, during which time I was tested for various suspects. I was even screened for a learning disability by a neurologist. All tests came back negative.

What followed was a very strange time. We'd spent the past decade working with a diagnosis of chronic Lyme disease, and yet this prestigious medical team dismissed out of hand the very mention of this supposed impossibility, demoting everything I felt was real into the mere conjurings of my imagination. This brush-off negated all we'd experienced up until that point, and, worse, the doctors' confidence in their opinion planted seeds of doubt in my own family. Even in myself.

I regularly visited my "renowned" psychiatrist, who concurred with my overseeing doctor that I was regressing. She believed I felt abandoned by my parents and wanted them to take care of me again, so I had fallen back to the symptoms they'd nursed me through during childhood, behaving like my younger, more dependent self. I didn't have the strength or confidence then to explain to her that my thoughts did not feel younger: they felt like they were aging by the second, struggling to traverse the war zone in my brain. But it wouldn't have mattered even if I could say something like that. Everyone believed I had no infectious disease; what authority did I have to say they were wrong?

And besides, what did I have to go on? What options did I have? These were my second, third, and fourth opinions consulted that fall. The conviction of so many experts in their fields ultimately shattered my faith in the validity of my own perspective. Things that once had felt certain became terrifyingly subjective. Fact became fiction; infectious disease became fabrication.

At the same time that I was losing trust in my own perceptions, my family lost faith in the physiological nature of my experience. I don't blame them for trusting in the authority of these doctors, but that doesn't change the fact that I felt completely isolated when they stopped believing there was a *physiological* cause to my pain. If everyone thought I was creating these symptoms via my own volition, then I could just as easily stop them—and stop burdening everyone else with them. I could no longer speak honestly to my doctors or to my family, terrified my perspective would be dismissed as delusional. This breakdown of trust was the most traumatic aspect of my illness.

My emotionally induced silence was compounded by my inability to communicate. I've since learned that Lyme patients experiencing neurological symptoms often lose the ability to articulate those symptoms. I wasn't just struggling to express myself: I also struggled to understand others. This inability to "correctly" perceive what another was trying to express made everything worse. So much of what people said, regardless of how it was intended, felt like an attack on my fragile consciousness. The

45

smallest things would set me off. For example, I remember going with my mom to pick up my brother Conor from school one afternoon. Sitting in the front seat, shielding my eyes from the sun, I made a negative comment about his new school. To this Conor said, "Allie, suck it up." A ball of anger hardened in my stomach. His sentence embodied what everyone around me felt. I didn't hear him telling me to snap out of my negative attitude; I heard him telling me to snap out of my sickness. Whipped to a fury, my anger retaliated in a visceral "FUCK you!"

Then I started to sob. I felt I was no longer a part of the family unit that had sustained me for so long, and I didn't understand why that support system was now completely lost to me. I felt dismissed and silenced by the people I needed the most. It seemed I was the only person willing to defend my reality—but as the number of people who saw what I saw dwindled, so did my confidence in my own perception. While I knew psychology was indeed contributing to my suffering, I couldn't believe my mind was the only thing in play.

Once I started the penicillin I slowly felt myself crawling back toward health. I could listen to music again, and could eat full meals, sitting with my family at dinner. I started to again think in full sentences. I felt like I was gaining control of my body and my brain, which for a while had felt almost completely lost to me.

But with improved cognitive abilities came a clearer sense of what I'd been dealing with. I was outraged by the way these physicians had treated us: that their prejudice—judging my condition before even meeting me—trumped everything else, reducing me from a human being struggling to keep afloat to nothing more than an example from a textbook. I had gone to them seeking validation and support, but their preemptory dismissal of Lyme had left me feeling they hadn't even given me the time of day.

No matter how much I theoretically should have trusted the expertise of well-respected doctors, in order to do as they asked—to accept that there were no spirochetes left in my body—I would need to also accept that every painful sensation I'd experienced over the previous four years had been a product of my imagination. I would have had to accept that the reason various medicines had dissipated my pain was only because I had convinced myself they would. I would have had to accept that my father at his sickest had experienced psychosomatic symptoms—and that I had subconsciously mimicked his experience. And, most painfully, I would have had to accept that losing the ability to do the things I loved most—reading, writing, acting, talking—was merely a psychological or psychosomatic response. I could not accept that. I also couldn't shake the feeling that their prejudice against Lyme had unduly influenced their diagnosis. Something felt seriously, physically wrong with my body. This was more than a psychological break.

When I received the results of the blood tests run that September, I thought back to the results I'd gotten from Dr. Raxlen just weeks before. I'd tested positive for *Borrelia burgdorferi*. Dr. Raxlen recorded my tests for *Bartonella* and *Babesia* as "indeterminable," meaning, though the disease is in one's system, there isn't a high enough concentration to register a positive result. My Boston tests strangely did not list the results of a *Borrelia burgdorferi* blood test, and noted my *Babesia* test as definitively negative. They never tested for *Bartonella.*

In the days that followed, I kept reflecting back on my experience working with Dr. Raxlen. His confidence that I had persistent Lyme or other co-infections continued to nag at me. I had heard about other neurological symptoms of late-stage Lyme disease—they sounded shockingly similar to my own. And the fact that my father's neurological symptoms had been similar didn't *necessarily* mean I had mimicked his. He'd also had CT scans and MRIs, and the surface of his brain had showed angry lesions, proof of biological infection, as no psychsomia can produce such physical tracks. But Dr. Raxlen and my new doctors weren't work-

47

ing together on this. They functioned in two separate worlds, and I could occupy only one at a time.

I felt the same way with my family sometimes, like I was living in a different world from theirs. At one point that fall my mother said that if we made no headway in Boston she'd think about sending me to the Mayo Clinic for further treatment and testing. I didn't understand what "Mayo Clinic" meant; I only heard that she planned to send me away, that she disdained my experience. I felt myself yelling without knowing what words came out of my mouth. My fear and distrust were so potent I was unable to hear that her suggestion actually validated my experience. Her apparent "siding" with these doctors felt like a shocking break in her unconditional support and trust. I realize now that for her it may actually have been a continuation of support. I doubt it was easy for my mom to come to terms with the concept that two full years of intravenous antibiotic treatment had been unnecessary, but maybe she saw that acceptance as an opportunity to set us on the right track. At the time however, as soon as it seemed like she didn't believe something was physically wrong with my body, it felt like she had given up on me. We spoke different languages then, ever wary of each other.

A scene in Andrew Solomon's book *Far from the Tree: Parents, Children, and the Search for Identity* describes a family with an autistic child named Cece. Though she was normally nonverbal, by the time she entered her teenage years Cece had spoken four times in her life, each time in complete, situationally appropriate sentences. In one of these instances, when her mother stood up to turn off the television Cece clearly said, "I want my TV."

It seems to me that to have a child totally incapable of language, while distressing, would at least be straightforward: she cannot understand you, and you cannot understand her. In Cece's case, however, it seemed as though she could occasionally understand her family, and they could occasionally understand her. Solomon writes: "You must remain agnostic while talking to Cece, aware that she may be picking up everything, or that your words may be gibberish to her."[42]

When successful communication became precious in my family, I wish we'd known to be agnostic. Had we been patiently mindful that others' perspectives are not necessarily our own, our anger and mistrust might not have slowed the healing process as much as it did. It's hard to describe our family dynamic during that time: simultaneously loving, supportive, and dismissive. Though well-intended, we were unable to fully accept, let alone talk about, the disease that forged our mutual experience. And the lack of open discussion unfortunately proved hurtful to each other.

By November I was able to properly communicate my dissatisfaction with the Boston contingent, my mom agreed to consult Dr. Raxlen about my developments since seeing him. We told him everything: the sudden neurological symptoms, the consideration that all my symptoms were psychosomatic, the seeming benefit of the penicillin, the fears about prolonged medical treatment—everything.

His reply restored the faith that I'd refused to completely relinquish: my understanding of my own body. And, in retrospect, it all seems so simple. "Allie, when you get stressed out, do you sometimes get a cold?" I nodded. "It's not that these psychological life events are *not* affecting you: I'm sure they did, I'm sure they are. You aren't a sociopath. But that doesn't mean that you're not also sick. It doesn't mean that you don't have Lyme—and it definitely doesn't mean that you can't get better."

Dr. Raxlen recommended we try a relatively new treatment: shots of a drug called Bicillin, a form of penicillin previously used to treat syphilis. The drug gets inserted into muscle, and as it's thick, the consistency of glue, painful going in. My dad, once again my nurse, administered my shots twice weekly. After a couple weeks we finally started to see real improvement. My speech normalized, my brain started to clear. In December

I was able to drive myself back to New York to start home tutoring, returning to Massachusetts regularly for the medication.

While I felt my physical health was stabilizing, I knew I needed help in emotionally processing what I'd endured. I couldn't bring myself to risk feeling victimized again by a psychologist, so instead I started visiting an energy healer twice a week to talk through my experience. She was also a registered nurse, and was able to help administer my shots when I couldn't travel back home. Though I wasn't completely healed, it felt like life was restarting.

I went back to school full-time in January of 2009, and did everything I could to keep my Boston experience in my rearview mirror. I wrote my college essay about how I did not want to be defined by the disease. I lied when my peers at school asked where I'd been during fall term. I fixated on my relationships with Heather and Calvin to distract myself from the tension of my strained family dynamic. I pulled away from my trauma, investing fully in a life separate from all things Lyme.

Of course I couldn't forget so easily. Every time I lay on my stomach to get my Bicillin shot, I heard doctors' voices telling me I wasn't sick. I'd imagine my mom nodding as they told me it was psychological; I'd hear my friends tell me it made sense, that I was just really freaked out about everything. While I wanted to say the Bicillin had definitely helped me, was it possible that what had actually helped was just my conviction that it would?

A doctor once shared a curious observation: as soon as many of his patients recovered enough to understand the truth of their experience with Lyme, their horror in what they'd endured triggered symptoms of post-traumatic stress disorder. While I won't equate my experience with PTSD, I do know that I created a mental block, a thick wall in my consciousness, behind which I imprisoned my memories of the fall of 2008. These would not see the light of day for almost four years.

CHAPTER 6

DIVISIONS

At my childhood home, a line of shadow split my front yard into two clean sections. If I arranged my body exactly on the line, my body split in half; I could feel the heat of the sun on one side of my face while the other remained cool, shielded from the light. I first did this when I was very young, maybe six or seven. I saved this two-tone shadow for myself, lying in its path only when I knew no one could see me.

My siblings indulged with me in the shadows, playing with division without ever realizing the game. My sister and I would lie in the shadows of the trees, finger-tracing the patterns of the branches on our skin. I kissed a boy for the first time in the shadow of those trees, as if we were hidden from sight.

Our house had a root cellar, an old building built into the side of a hill. Its roof was always warm, lit by the sun, but its stone walls were shielded, and so were always cool. Even in summer that shadow space was refreshing, its temperature lower, the grass wet. Standing on top of the root cellar, I could look down one story below me into that shadow space; and if I jumped off the hot roof I fell from sun into shade, the temperature dropping with me. It was like jumping into another world.

One afternoon I dared Conor to jump, jumping first to show him he could do it. I remember looking back up at the roof; the way the sun shone from behind him I could hardly see his face. It was as if he were held by the above world when I jumped into the other, that we could no longer coexist. I didn't anticipate his jump into my world, and when he landed he cried. I don't know whether his tears were from pain or from fear, but I was convinced I could stop them if I could find a way to fuse his world of light with my world of shadow.

In the months and years following 2008, I no longer felt capable of straddling worlds, existing in half light, half shadow. Desperate to separate myself from the events consumed by Lyme disease, I quarantined in my consciousness everything that had brought me pain, and instead tried to nurture the parts of myself that had survived the onslaught. In the fall of 2009 I started my freshman year at Bard College, in Annandale-on-Hudson, New York. I saw college as a fresh start, a brilliant opportunity to redefine myself as someone free from the burden and pain of a misunderstood disease. I stepped ever forward, trying fervently to not look back.

Of course, it was impossible to completely erase that time in my life. Though I rarely spoke about it, my friends at Bard knew vaguely what had happened. Calvin was my only friend who had lived through my illness, and he was my greatest support in helping me live beyond it. He honored my need to move forward as though I were unaffected, and held my hand when I found myself traveling back, trapped in my memories. I worked to visit the past as infrequently as possible, and obsessed instead over my present and future.

For a long time this technique seemed to work. I had a small flare-up during the spring of my freshman year, but that was as easily stopped with another course of antibiotics as it was brushed under the carpet. The Lyme that had been so horribly stubborn for the prior five years finally seemed under control. I left it behind.

Or so I had thought. The day before I started my senior year of college, I pulled out from under my bed a box that held old photo albums and other keepsakes. I flipped through an album of Calvin and me at his senior prom in spring of 2008, smiling to myself at how happy we looked, how blissfully ignorant we were about what was soon to come. At the end of the album was a single loose picture. Heather had taken it on the first day of my senior year of high school, exactly four years earlier. I'm standing on the steps of our house in Katonah, smiling alone into the camera. The front door is open behind me, and if you look closely you can see the nearly empty living room and bare walls of the house we would squat in that year.

I took out the picture and faced the mirror, looking back and forth between the picture and my reflection. At first I could hardly see a difference. My face was the same shape. My eyes were the same color. Though my hair was shorter in the mirror, and my cheeks more full, I still looked like the person smiling back at me from four years earlier.

I took another look in the mirror and then closed my eyes, focusing instead on what I looked like inside. I searched for pain, but felt nothing but a little stiffness in my neck. I opened my palms on my knees, and felt the entirety of my hands on the entirety of my knees—with no sensory dropouts like bad radio reception. I wiggled my toes. I smiled. Everything moved without a glitch. Then I opened my eyes to look again at the photograph. I saw how I had held my shoulders up slightly, tension pulling them toward my ears. I saw how tight my teeth looked in my smile, as if they were bearing against some kind of pain. My hair was thinner, exhausted. What at first glance looked similar was after scrutiny an entirely different space. My body, which was once so dangerous, now felt safe, and which was once so weak, now seemed strong.

I pitied myself then, attempting to create a further barrier between the person in the picture and the person in the mirror—but I couldn't do it. Looking at myself in the mirror, I could see that everything I had pushed away was still inside me. The girl in the mirror and the girl in the picture were the same. I would never be able to wish away the trauma of my senior year of high school. It defined me, no matter how much I didn't want to admit it.

My efforts to block so many formative events and interactions from my memory had fragmented my identity. Once those memories started to resurface, they kept on coming. Bits of conversations, flashes of pain filled my consciousness. I collected them all, trying to piece together the shattered images, sensations, and sounds too long suppressed.

When I was sick, other than with my dad, I didn't seek community with others who shared my experience—even at the IV clinics, when I was surrounded by patients suffering the same illness. I broke my identity into pieces, occupying the ugly bits only when it was absolutely necessary. But now that I was reflecting back, examining the returned stray pieces, I found myself wondering how different things might have been if I had talked to people who understood intimately what I was going through. Were there such people? I'd always known there must be, but never before had I needed to find them.

The thought of my history being unavoidably part of a larger shared experience of chronic Lyme disease, or of chronic disease in general, terrified me. I didn't want there to exist an environment where the feelings of shame I had faced, the struggle for acceptance, was normal, where others felt the same. I didn't want anyone to feel the prejudice I had felt when my symptoms continued past the date it was decided they would stop. As strongly as I felt this, I also knew many others suffer as I suffered—and not just from the disease, but also, maybe more so, from the entrenched medical and social inability to accept that disease. With that realization came an intense desire to learn more about the 10 to 20 percent of people whose symptoms of Lyme persist. If there was a shared chronic Lyme narrative, I wanted to find it. I probably needed to find it.

PART II

VOICES BEYOND THE WALL

I once met a woman whose breath came quickly in her chest, her feet tread lightly on the ground. Though her movements seemed charged with a nervous energy, she looked normal, healthy even. But she told me she felt a thick glass wall separated her from the rest of the world. She could see and hear what was going on around her, but no one could hear her; nothing she said penetrated that glass. Later she reached out and touched me with a hand that was clammy and cold. Though my first instinct was to pull away, I instead held her hand in mine. When we let go, I noticed a new lightness in her, and realized that my small gesture had forged a crack in her wall.

In 2012 and 2013 I conducted a series of interviews with many chronic Lyme patients in an attempt to better understand others experience chronic Lyme disease. I set out to discover to what degree my own experience had been an anomaly. I also wanted to offer fellow sufferers my ears, my attention; more so, I wanted to offer them a respect for their experience that I at times had been desperate for myself. I wanted to give voice to others who've also felt silenced by our medical system.

In the following interviews, all names have been changed to protect the identities of the brave patients who shared their experiences with me—as well as of the doctors who helped save their lives.

CHAPTER 7

A SAFE SPACE

"Thank you all for coming. I know it's not easy for you guys to get out here every Thursday night, and I thank you for that." She had a soothing voice, the kind that could lull you to sleep if she spoke quietly enough. "What I want to do is quickly go around the circle and have you introduce yourselves, giving a short synopsis of your story—only if you feel comfortable, of course." She anchored her gaze on mine. "I see some new faces here. I'll go first."

To be honest, my preconceived notions of Lyme support groups have always been negative. Imagining a group of sick people talking about their pain didn't seem particularly attractive to me. The only way I knew how to deal with illness was to push through it, so I'd always preferred spending time with healthy friends rather than talking about disease. It felt like wallowing, which seemed dangerously stagnant to me. Of course, this judgment of mine was not unlike the judgment of people outside the Lyme community. For a long time I thought we all should buck up, stop talking, start doing.

But then again, I came to realize this sharing was actually a form of doing. The simple idea that my own experience might be a part of larger narrative or phenomenon fueled my desire to better understand it. After having pushed away this part of my life for so long, I wanted to finally try to come to terms with my experience by immersing myself in the world of illness once again—to surround myself with people who intimately knew what it meant to live with Lyme disease.

When I arrived at my first meeting, the church was dark. All of the doors were locked. Looking for a way inside, I wandered around the perimeter. I was struck by the simplicity of the church, so unlike the elaborate or glamorous Catholic churches I was used to. It looked a school, or a doctor's office; free of pride or decoration, the simple brick building didn't try to prove itself. This lack of presumption made me feel out of place.

I found the meeting at the end of a hall, where seven people sat quietly around a single table, seeking sanctuary in a community of their own creation. I had come to take part as a silent observer, to collect their stories and then to leave. But by the end of the meeting I found myself moved by conversations I'd once rolled my eyes about. Drawn toward the sense of community there, I returned multiple times. And each time I was a bit in awe of how those who spoke knew their story would help another person sitting at the table. In the acknowledgment of shared experiences, personal stories became single chapters in a much bigger storybook. In this circle, chronic Lyme was seen as a global phenomenon, one that was further validated in the telling of each story.

Our facilitator, Irene Billings, shared first. She had been infected with Lyme disease in 1970 when she was clearing a wooded area behind her home in Charlotte, North Carolina. Hers was one of the earliest cases detected outside of Lyme, Connecticut. It started with a rash that was diagnosed as poison ivy, except that the rash didn't go away. She sought medical treatment for the sickness she felt overtaking her body, but no doctor understood what was going on. She was hospitalized for twenty days, during which time she was tested for a number of illnesses. "It looked like an autoimmune disease, they told me. I remember sitting in my hospital gown after my second hospital admission, and my doctor telling me—'I know something is wrong, but I just can't find it.'"

In the absence of a definitive diagnosis, Irene started to assume that something about her psyche was making her sick. All of her friends believed she was suffering from some kind of mental issue—and, eventually, so did she. She had always been healthy, energetic, and optimistic, but she'd since become overwhelmed with a myriad of symptoms of depression. After months of illness, she and her family moved to Hudson Valley, where she started treatment for her depression.

"It's not that I wasn't depressed," she said. "Of course I was depressed. I was sick and nobody could help me. But the only thing they would do was put me on antidepressants. This was the 1970s—they do the same thing now." Then another doctor diagnosed her with systemic lupus, and her mood elevators and antidepressants were halted in favor of high-dose anti-inflammatories and beta-blockers.

After nearly nine years, her mind started to fail her, her body barely functioning. "My husband couldn't deal with it," she told the group, recounting the story of losing her marriage to the pressures of chronic illness. The trajectory of her downward spiral got a jolt, however, when she started reading about Lyme disease, and found the description of its telltale rash.

Now, almost forty years later, thanks to extensive medical intervention and patience, Irene considers herself healthy. And for the last ten years she's hosted this group to help those like her. "Unfortunately, many others have fallen through the cracks with undiagnosed Lyme disease. I know how sick you can feel, and how frustrating it can be to bear it alone. I may not have all the answers for you, but I want to hear you. I don't know if the antibiotics really helped after so long. Perhaps the Lord healed me, or maybe my body figured out how to deal with it. I do know that God gave me grace, and that is why I am here today, speaking with all of you." With that, she nodded her head, and said a silent prayer to herself. Then she turned to her left and motioned for the next person to start. Halfway around the circle, a frail woman took a small notepad from her bag and rested a pen above it. As we went around the table introducing ourselves, she wrote down each name, as if she feared forgetting each new name she heard.

"My name is Peter," he said into his lap. "I'm not ready to share my story today." The two people after him declined as well. I could see on Irene's face that she prayed for each of them as their turn passed by.

The next woman to speak was very fragile. The way she sat in her chair: her feet hovered just above the floor, as if just touching its surface would be too much contact. She wore loose clothes. I'd noticed earlier that she shook no one's hand. But behind her papery skin and tired eyes I could see a fire searching for any oxygen it could find, fighting to regain its strength. When she introduced herself her voice wavered, as if her own name didn't seem familiar to her anymore.

"In 2008, I woke up with a jaw ache that I thought had to be the flu." We laughed knowingly. "Days passed though, and it didn't seem to go away. My partner insisted I go to the doctor, so to appease her I promised I would. I, of course, did not have the flu. The doctor told me I had Lyme disease. I remember thinking to myself, Lyme disease? Don't you get that from hiking or something?" We laughed again. She was prescribed the traditional three weeks of doxy, and her jaw ache disappeared. Cured. But, of course, the tightness in her jaw returned a couple of months later, along with strange aches and pains she attributed to menopause. "I remember what adolescence was like," she giggled, "and everything was so crazy back then. It didn't seem too strange that things would be just as crazy on this end too." But as the years passed she started to notice a numbness in her hands. This time we did not laugh. "I was convinced I had multiple sclerosis — it's in my family, see. When I went back to the doctor, they diagnosed me with diabetes, but something about that seemed strange to me. I'm underweight if anything, and I never had problems like that before."

She continued diabetes treatment for a full year—change of diet, exercise, blood sugar monitoring and insulin injections—without seeing any improvement. The only thing that helped her was massage. One day her massage therapist confided that she questioned the diabetes diagnosis: her son had diabetes, and she knew the symptoms well. "Isn't it funny?" our fellow sufferer said to us, "How all we need is one stranger to validate our thought processes, and the world seems easier to walk through again?" The massage therapist thought it still might be Lyme, and recommended a specialist in the area. "He was famous, she told me, for helping people with Lyme."

In her first meeting with the doctor, she told him about a recent vaginal infection she'd had that neither her gynecologist nor emergency room doctors had answers for. The pain from that treasured part of her was so intense that she felt separated from her own sexuality—and from her own personality—in almost every way. It was an incredibly personal confession, one that made her blush as she spoke it.

"I asked him, could it be Lyme? And he spent a couple minutes making jokes about me. Mean jokes, inappropriate jokes, sexual jokes that I will not repeat. I want to maintain my sense of dignity in this group." This supposed expert belied his reputation as one who saved Lyme patients from the doctors who did not understand them. Fortunately, after years of misdiagnosis, a spinal tap later confirmed our friend suffered from Lyme, and she never looked back.

It was only as she closed her story, telling us she was seeing a nurse practitioner a friend had recommended, that she finally lifting her gaze from her notepad to make eye contact with us. "I like her a lot," she said. "The first time I went, I opened the door and there were people sitting in lawn chairs getting IVs in the basement. I love that. It feels pioneering. I don't feel judged. I can't tell if it's the safety and acceptance or the medicine that is saving my life, but I'm thankful for it either way."

I thought about my own basement clinic, and how much I ultimately resented it. I hoped she wouldn't come to feel that way, and that she wouldn't need IV in a lawn chair long enough to yearn for something new.

When she stopped speaking silence again flooded the room, and I realized the attention had settled on me. This was the first time I was asked to share my experience with people outside of my personal or medical life. I told a condensed version of my story. I did not share my own doubts about the disease, or the fear that my doctors had by then engrained in me. I played the part of my peers. I spoke with authority, certain that I suffered from a chronic illness and not from a psychiatric disorder. As I spoke, I realized my audience seemed to believe my story. I noticed, too, that for the first time my words flowed easily off my tongue.

The woman sitting to my left, Bridget had the last turn, and she readily filled most of our remaining half hour with her voice. Without a single hand gesture except the occasional touch to her hair, she spoke with great authority. "Think about a firefly," she said. "When you try to catch one, the fear and stress of being caught creates a physical reaction in the insect. It starts blinking, faster and faster. Sometimes it dies. That's what happened to me, I started blinking so fast I almost died."

She was regal, yet without ornamentation. Something about her energy dominated the room, and she had a comfortable self-confidence that none of us could match. "I had no doubt I had Lyme as soon as I showed any symptoms," she said firmly. She sat straight in her chair, her hands comfortably in her lap, and she looked around the table, continually making eye contact with each of us as she spoke. "I was working at the Omega Institute in June of 2011 when I found a tick on my thigh." She told us that at Omega, a holistic studies education center, they were asked to not remove ticks on their own—to instead go straight to the nurse, which she did. At the health center her attendant looked at the tick and said, "Well, let's just see if you get sick"—without removing the tick. About a week and a half later, Bridget returned with vertigo and a high fever. They released her saying she had a cold. Bridget looked around the room again. Her gaze landed on me as she said, "I don't know how I didn't die." I looked away, too embarrassed to return her gaze.

Seeking help outside the institute, she quickly found a doctor who diagnosed Lyme and prescribed four weeks of doxycycline. She felt well for two full weeks after the treatment, but then got sick again. Only then, eight weeks after her bite, did she finally remove the tick from her leg. When she told us that, at first I wondered why she hadn't taken off the tick herself—but then quickly looked down into my lap. I didn't want to doubt her; doubt was what I was trying to fight against. As a kind of punishment to myself, I didn't form my thoughts into a question. She then introduced a new doctor into her story, "the anarchist," who refused to treat her even though she tested positive on every test. She attributed his refusal to the hysteria he projected onto her.

"In 1975 I watched my house burn down. My sister and father died inside. The doctor attributed my symptoms, my seizures and my hallucinations, to PTSD. Antibiotics wouldn't help me, he said. I needed to deal with the psychological issues that were the apparent bedrock of my experience." Bridget assured us she had already dealt with her PTSD. As I listened to her story, I couldn't get her doctor's hypothesis out of my mind. "I went two years without treatment," she told us. "I had no insurance, no money, I was homeless, and was forced to go to my family for support. I remember praying to God: just take me. That's it. I'm done."

I shifted uncomfortably in my seat. Why couldn't I empathize with this woman? I had marveled at people's ability to persist through that pain without judgment. Why, now, did I fail? Trapped in my own head, I tried to break free from my own consciousness, judging my thoughts as soon as they occurred to me. That sense of oneness I had felt at the table was dissipating, and I was desperate to get it back.

"I knew then that no one else would help me, so I had to help myself. I told myself that I was just a host: that concept enabled me to understand I needed to fight a war. It wasn't going to be a violent war; this was about strategy. I needed to understand what the spirochetes needed, and how they survived—and then I needed to take that away from them." She outlined every type of sugar and every type of meat that spirochetes fed on. She described the way they burrow into our muscle tissue, and the way they protect themselves by forming cysts and spores, which antibiotics can't penetrate. She spoke with pride about how she had conquered her elusive enemy. "I'm not sick anymore. And I know now that there is a gift in Lyme. It gave me a connection to a high power. I'm a better person for it."

Her story was eerily reminiscent of a doctor I'd had in 2007 at the Life Extension Center, a clinic that offered alternative, holistic medical care for patients with chronic and degenerative diseases. Though many patients began their treatment journey there, many others came only after exhausting all other treatment options. A close friend of my family named Kate started treatment for her breast cancer at the clinic; there she received high-dose intravenous vitamin C so as to supercharge her immune system into fighting the cancer on its own. She had recommended I visit the Life Extension Center with the hope that I might turn my own chronic condition into a cured one.

At the Life Extension Center, my doctor had also described fighting the disease in terms of battle strategy. We needed to starve the enemy of its sustenance, and work to boost the strength and energy of my immune system's army to aid in attack. He started my treatment by stripping my diet of as many sugars as possible, as sugar fuels the spirochetes' fire. I couldn't eat any meat, dairy, carbohydrates, processed sugars, raw sugars, or caffeine. I was limited to a small list of fruits and vegetables. My mother added brown rice to that list, but we both knew that was cheating. The diet was complimented by a nutrient cocktail intended to be the consistency of a milkshake, but it was actually mixed into powdery milk, which smelled of vomit. I was asked to drink sixteen ounces of this three times daily. If I couldn't keep it down, I was to make some more and drank it again. This was the weapon I used to fight my battle.

Strangely, when it came time to boost my immune system, my support system would mysteriously disappear. Everyone cleared out of the kitchen after my mother mixed the drink for me, leaving me to swallow my battle fuel on my own. Though they'd occasionally call out if they thought I needed something, it was always from a safe distance. Forcing down my slop on my own, vulnerable without my armor of antibiotics, I felt even more alone.

Another weapon in my Life Extension arsenal was the same vitamin-C drip that Kate was using to treat her cancer. For this, I went to the clinic three times a week for the first few months of my junior year, always sitting next to an elderly cancer patient. As his nurse brought him from his residence in assisted living, I imagined it was the highlight of his day. At the time I was working on a production of *The Comedy of Errors*; he knew the play well enough to randomly recite lines during our time together, which always made me smile. Sometimes my mom and I would sing to pass the time, and his foot would tap along to her tune, as if she were singing directly to him. Even in the midst of cancer treatment, this man was able to find joy, and share it.

His face started to turn gray about two months into my own treatment, and I knew it was time for him to go. He stopped coming to the Life Extension Center before my mom and I had even learned his name, and we never saw him again. I cried at his assumed death in a way that I had never cried about death before. I hated the fact that I was gaining strength at the same time that this joyous man was losing his.

A woman who seemed burdened by the world filled the seat he'd left. When she wasn't fighting with her children over the phone, she'd harangue us about the conspiracy theories she'd discovered in her short experience with the medical system. Though she hated life as much as her predecessor had loved it, cancer chose no sides, and mutated both of their bodies with equal prejudice.

One time, while listening to this young woman rant beside me, I remember looking at my mother and thinking how lucky I was to have faced this sickness with the support I had. Up until that point my doctors had treated me well, our insurance company had covered my treatment, my school had accommodated my illness, and my friends and family had always loved me, fiercely. I was tremendously lucky, and my luck continued.

The IV successfully boosted my immune system into fighting the spirochetes on its own. For the first time in years I was able to survive without antibiotics. With the color that came back to my skin, I barely recognized my face in the mirror. I'd wake up in the morning with energy instead of pain. My mind was clear, and every day I looked forward to walking through the hallways at school. I felt good. So good, in fact, that I decided to stop treatment. What I didn't know.

Back at the support group, I looked up at Bridget, who returned my gaze immediately as if she'd known my attention had wandered and she'd been waiting for me to reengage. A young boy, who'd declined to share his story, raised his hand. "So the medicine I'm on now," he asked, "you don't think it's going to help me?"

"No," she said. "Not at all." The boy didn't speak again. She judged him with a prejudice from the other side, the side of the sick who, left with nothing, are forced to fend for themselves. I realized then that my discomfort with her wasn't about the truth of her story, but about its agenda. In the support group we were aiming to support each other, but it seemed she came just to have us support her, offering none in return.

Though she perturbed me, she also enlightened me. As relieved as I was to discover a living chronic Lyme narrative at that church, I also quickly realized the articulation of that narrative was imperfect. My perspective—like Bridget's, or even Irene's—may be flawed, and thus easy to dismiss on its own. But if enough voices and perspectives came together, and our collective stories told a singular message, maybe our perspective would be harder to dismiss. If enough people communicated the same thought in the same moment, wouldn't it be an act of ignorance to turn away?

To build that symphony of voices, telling a similar story so loud it would be impossible to ignore, I started searching for fellow sufferers willing to share their experiences of chronic Lyme. I posted flyers in doctor's offices, I sent emails to everyone I knew, and I hoped word of mouth would reach those I didn't know how to find. Given how I had for years been unwilling to speak about my own experience, I was initially worried no one would be willing to talk with me. I soon discovered I was very wrong.

CHAPTER 8

MELISSA EDWARDS

Melissa, twenty-four, saw a flyer I had posted in her doctor's office. She was living in New York City at the time, so I met her in person in a private room at the New York Public Library. Her energy was calm and settled, and though at times it seemed as difficult for her to verbalize her story as it was for me to hear it, she also seemed freed by the process.

To follow are excerpts from her interview transcript.

Of course my mind always wonders: Where did I get it? How did I get it? Why did I get it? But I consider myself fairly lucky because I haven't had a lifelong struggle. I was always a healthy kid. I graduated from college. I went back home to Tennessee and realized that not everyone got to live the life I led.

Then I woke up one morning and I had this rash. I didn't know what it was. I went to the doctor that I grew up with—I played soccer with his daughter for ten years, so they were like family—he told me that he thought I had a spider bite, gave me some cream, but didn't give me any antibiotics. So I thought, okay it's a spider bite, but then almost exactly one month later I started having this kind of brain fog. I couldn't see clearly. I couldn't focus on driving. In the middle of the night, I would wake up with my heart rate at 150 and this horrible pain up the back of my scalp. I felt like a knife was stabbing my kneecap. Every joint on the left side of my body felt like it was on fire. Something had to be very wrong. I discovered Lyme through internet research and thought maybe I had it. I had a bite. I had a rash. It didn't seem like rocket science to me.

I went back to that small-town doctor to talk about Lyme, and I left the appointment crying. I was screaming. He told me I couldn't have Lyme, that I needed anti-depressants, and that there was nothing he could do for me. All the symptoms were in my head. I remember my mom was whispering to me across the room to take the prescription for the anti-depressants. "We don't have to take it," she mouthed to me.

"No." I looked him right in the eyes and said, "I'm not taking this. I'm not crazy." I think that was the turning point for me. It could have gone a whole different way. As I was leaving, his wife, my old soccer coach, came out to talk to me. She told me that her husband was an expert on Lyme disease in the area, and that it was not possible that I had it. I knew something was wrong with me. I'm not crazy. I was perfectly healthy a few months back, and then I couldn't move.

My mother found an infectious disease doctor that I could go and see. We went to Nashville to see this lady who apparently knew Lyme very well, and when we got there I told her everything that had happened. Back then, it seemed like my story was already long. "You weren't given any antibiotics when you had the rash?" she asked. "If you have a rash, if you have a bite, and you start feeling bad, it's obvious what it is." I remember yelling, "Thank you!" I found somebody who will help me. She ran a bunch of blood work and everything came back negative except one band on the Western blot test. It was band 41 and it came back positive. She told me I didn't have enough positive bands to be considered positive for Lyme. "There is nothing else I can do for you."

I left her office at the lowest of the lows. The symptoms kept getting worse. I would sit at a restaurant and a shooting pain would go down my spine. I would scream and think, nobody understands. I couldn't control what was going on.

We finally found this one ILADS [International Lyme and Associated Diseases Society] doctor, but had to travel to Mississippi to see him. His office was this little building in the middle of a cotton field, five hours away from my house. It looked decrepit, but I think it saved my life. I tested negative again, but he trusted my symptoms and prescribed me high-dose oral antibiotics. Finally I started to feel better. It was working very quickly until I reached a point that it didn't work anymore. I realized then that it was time to go to New York. There was just nobody in Tennessee who would believe me. They don't listen and they don't believe you, because apparently Lyme in the South is unheard of. The ticks don't stop at the state line. It was just ridiculous. I knew there would be many more resources for me when I got to New York. I had to go.

Once I made it here, I met with a doctor who told me that I not only had Lyme but also *Babesia*, and possibly *Bartonella*. I burst into tears in his office, just in relief. After a few months in New York I had gotten a little bit better, but my neurological symptoms weren't going away. It hit me one day, all of a sudden, I couldn't speak like I used to. The things I said didn't make any sense. I felt the biggest effects in my nervous system. I remember a time when I could speak in front of hundreds of people and never get nervous. Now, I'll be watching a commercial and think, "Oh my gosh, what's going to happen next?" My heart rate jumps, I can't control anything. I keep looking for stories of people who get better, about people who don't have to suffer with this for their whole lives. I'm prepared to cope with this for a couple of years, but I just can't accept that I'm going to be stuck like this. Right now, I have to focus on having a life that's livable. I want something more than that.

It's only been a year and a half for me, and when I learn about other people who have dealt with this disease, it seems like it hasn't been too bad. Nobody in my family ever told me I was wrong, or to stop what I was doing—and good thing too because, to be frank, I would have died. They were always behind me. That said, it's hard for people to really understand what this is actually like. I can't go to the park. I can't go to the movies. I just can't do it. People just don't understand. None of them have ever said to my face we don't believe you, this is ridiculous, but I don't think they will ever be able to comprehend what this is like for me. I don't think anyone can unless they've experienced it themselves.

The people who have been the least supportive of me are those in the medical field, ironically. So many of them tell you that they understand you better than you do. I go to this walk-in clinic to get a shot three times a week. Each time I see a different doctor I have to explain my situation. "These are prescribed to me," I tell them. "I pick them up at the pharmacy, they are covered by insurance, please administer the shot." Every time the doctors say, "Who is prescribing this to you? Where are you getting these drugs?" They talk like I'm some sort of criminal. I see people getting shots when diagnosed with other diseases without a problem. The biggest problem is that I can't give them my doctor's name. People always tell me, "Do not give the doctor's name," because insurance companies will contact them or try and take their license away if they find out they're prescribing more than is technically recommended to treat Lyme, like the Bicillin shots. I've even gotten to the point to where I've learned not to tell people I have it. When I started applying for jobs, I told them why I had been out of work for a year and they looked at me with disgust. I can't tell anyone the truth about my life anymore. It's just depressing.

But I've been lucky because I never believed that I was disgusting, or crazy, or that my doctors were crazy. I always believed I had something that could be fixed. See, I have a friend in Massachusetts who went the hospital with symptoms of Lyme disease. They didn't treat her. No. They put her in a psych ward. For four years she was on psych medication, when all she needed was an antibiotic to treat her Lyme disease. I also know a boy from my town in Tennessee who was experiencing symptoms and I told him to speak up. "You have to tell them to test for Lyme," I told him, "and don't believe them if it comes back negative." He did, he got treatment, and now he's better. It can go either way, and we just have to speak up so that people can get better. It's just amazing that just people talking to each other is what's changing this.

I've really come a ways because of it. I'm not in bed anymore. I'm trying to get a part-time job. I still have this anxiety about my heart rate because I feel like it controls me. I have to take my beta-blocker everywhere with me. I used to live on the sixth floor of a walk-up and there were two times that I thought I was definitely going to die. My heart was going so fast when I walked up the stairs; I could feel it everywhere. At one point I had 911 dialed on my phone and I remember thinking to myself, "There is nobody here. I'm going to die on the fifth floor and nobody's here." It's just so depressing to think about.

Even as a little kid, I couldn't imagine anything worse than an illness. It would always frustrate me when people weren't grateful for their health. I was a healthy child, and I was like, Why do I feel like this? One day this is going to come back to me. People really take their health for granted.

It's just so important for me to get people more aware of this. Because like I said, talking to people is saving me. I mean that is everything. When nobody in your family has had it, you don't know anybody in town that's ever had it, doctors are telling you that you don't have it, just finding somebody that says, "I understand," can save your life.

Age used to matter to me so much, money was never important to me, I didn't care where I lived, but I always thought that by the time I'm a certain age maybe I'll be happy in the job I'm at, maybe I'll be married, or have children. Now none of that matters. It only matters that I'm healthy, and I get to a point where I can make enough to survive. So my outlook is completely changed, for the better I think. Success to me doesn't mean what it used it mean. This outlook keeps my idea of happiness keyed to something that is reachable, that's right here, today. I don't have to have something by the time I'm thirty or whatever. It doesn't matter anymore. It just matters that I'm alive. And I am—alive.

CHAPTER 9

CHARLOTTE LERMAN

Charlotte Lerman, fifty-one, was introduced to me by one of my closest friends from high school. Though she was from my town, Charlotte had moved to Arizona by the time we spoke. At one point during a conversation about arranging a phone interview, Charlotte said, "Anything I can do to help the cause." I hadn't yet realized a chronic Lyme cause even existed.

The following is drawn from my notes of our phone interview.

I was twenty-nine. Geez, when was that? 1990, I guess. My son was born in '92, so that makes me fifty-one years old now, if you can imagine that. At first I was told it was probably my wisdom teeth, because I was having these horrible head and neck aches. I was living in London at the time and went to see a couple of doctors about it, but I never felt helped or heard by them. I decided to have my wisdom teeth taken out in the hopes that my symptoms were as a result of them. There was a brief period of time when I was feeling better because I was being treated with antibiotics for the extraction, but two weeks after surgery the headaches and pain were back. Obviously the pain was not a result of my teeth.

It was months before anyone told me about Lyme. My husband's associate had it and, based on what he knew and had researched, he diagnosed me over the phone saying that it was probably what I had. He was the one that recommended I see someone that knew about Lyme. He gave me the name of his specialist to go and see. I was hopeful of course, but had no real idea if that was what I had.

I traveled back to the States to see this doctor. He knew I had waited months to see him and that I had been recommended by one of his patients. I did not test positive for Lyme or any other co-infection, but the doctor told me that I had such a high number of Lyme symptoms that he was willing to treat me even though I did not have a positive test result. At the time, this was a big risk for him as a doctor. He kept trying to tell me I was lucky to have found him. I kept wondering, *I have thirty-six out of the forty symptoms on your checklist. How could you not treat me?* He did treat me continuously for nine months, with oral and IV treatment, until I found out I was pregnant.

It was my third pregnancy. I showed up to my OB-GYN with a PICC line for my IV antibiotics in my arm and I remember him saying, "Please don't tell me you're pregnant." I told him I was and that I had Lyme, but he did not know much about Lyme and pregnancy. He showed me this two-paragraph-long article that was years old, and asked me what I wanted him to do. I wanted to follow the advice of my specialist, and stay on antibiotics through the pregnancy. Based on the information he knew however, he told me he couldn't recommend that. I told him that based on what I knew I wanted to stay on the drugs and that he could consult with my Lyme specialist regarding treatment.

I had spoken to a woman that had given birth to twins and had to watch them die after she had gone to her OB-GYN with a Lyme rash on her face and her doctor told that she didn't need to be treated. That woman strongly recommended staying on the antibiotics, as did my Lyme specialist. Everyone I knew hung on to every word of their OB-GYN, but I knew it was going to be different for me when my doctor told me I needed to go off antibiotics during my pregnancy. That scared me. I was finally feeling better. I couldn't take steps back. What if I gave it to the baby? I knew then that I had to use my voice or I was going to die, or worse, I was going to kill my child.

Young moms spend days looking for the right doctor during pregnancy. I did the same, but I wasn't looking for someone to make me feel happy and comfortable—I was looking for someone willing to give me the medicine I knew I needed. Ultimately, I took the advice of the Lyme specialist who agreed to treat me in conjunction with my OB-GYN and asked if I was willing to have post-birth testing of the placenta and my child. I maintained constant treatment of oral amoxicillin during all nine months to keep the infection at bay and to protect my unborn child. The treatment was a success. I gave birth to a healthy boy, who has never showed any signs of the disease.

But I was lucky. I know women who haven't been so lucky. A friend of mine had five miscarriages after two very normal pregnancies, never knowing the miscarriages were probably due to her Lyme. Even after she was diagnosed and treated she had three more miscarriages before she adopted her daughter. Another friend of mine was infected and treated for Lyme and still suffered through three miscarriages before she was able to have a child. A tick bit her, she had the ring, but the doctor refused to put her on antibiotics while she was pregnant. Seven months later she gave birth to twins. Both children died on different days, several days after their births. In their autopsies, they tested off-the-charts positive for Lyme, *Bartonella*, and *Babesia*. The tick killed them. How many women do you think have lost babies because of Lyme disease?

After my placenta was biopsied, it was determined that there were spirochetes present within it. The results were written up by my doctor in an effort to prove that spirochetes can live in the body after extended antibiotic treatment. Not much has come from it. My son was never treated with antibiotics because he had no signs of the disease, but after his birth he was tested for two years. As an adolescent he got a tick bite and developed a rash. Of course I insisted he get treated, and thankfully he's never had any long-term issues with this disease.

It just drives me insane. No one seems to buy this. Both my brother-in-law and brother are doctors, and at the time neither of them believed that Lyme could cause all the symptoms that I was having. What did they think? I was making it up? I have a fine relationship with them now, but they just weren't aware then, like so many doctors are still not aware now. What is it about this disease that turns people off? I still haven't figured it out. It's been thirty years.

My son is healthy. That's what matters. And I'm mostly healthy. I don't think I have the disease active in my system anymore, but I can still feel some of the residual, leftover damage. One of the most difficult symptoms I deal with are these full-body seizures. No one seems to be able to figure out what sets them off, and I stay conscious throughout them. The strangest thing is that they don't reregister on any machine. I'll be flopping around like a fish and it doesn't show up anywhere. I guess we don't have the technology to measure them or something. Makes you feel like it's all in your head though. Sometimes, not always of course, but sometimes.

Just never underestimate what this disease can do to you. It will attack the weakest part of you, and the only thing you can do is speak up and hope someone will listen. Find someone who will put themselves on the line for you. You'll need it.

INTERLUDE

After my interview with Charlotte I felt saddened, and hoped that her experience had been simply a product of her time. Unfortunately, this was not the case. I found at least four studies published in major medical journals warning of the effect of Lyme during pregnancy. In 1983, "Borrelia-like spirochetes" were found on a neonatal blood smear. Just two years later in 1985, neonatal death was recorded with Borrelia in the infant's spleen, bone marrow, and myocardium. The bacteria had infiltrated the most complex biological systems in the infant, and were reproducing inside the infant's bones, a nearly impossible place to treat infection. Two more Borrelia-related deaths were recorded in the years following; the first official record of Lyme-caused neonatal death was filed in 1988.[43] *Charlotte's fears had been studied and well-documented for almost a decade before her pregnancy, and yet she, and the other women in her story, struggled to find doctors who would give them the treatment Charlotte correctly believed was necessary. Had she not "used her voice" as she had, her boy might have been another study statistic.*

A quick Google search of children who have died from Lyme reveals disturbing images of cold, stiff, empty bodies. The emaciated babies had been unable to fully develop before the bacteria overpowered them. These children were dead before they had a chance to be born.

CHAPTER 10

JUDY REAGAN

The following transcript derives from an interview conducted in the library of the high school where Judy Reagan, sixty-one, works as the librarian. Soon after I arrived at the school library, we were placed under lockdown in response to a gun threat. No one could enter or leave the library. Under the circumstances I expected to postpone our interview, but Judy insisted we press on, though she did periodically pause our conversation to check on her students and ensure everyone was safe. We sat at a table in the back of the room. Even though we were somewhat isolated and trapped, her story, told mostly in an intense whisper, nonetheless transported me back into the complex world of chronic illness, a place I always had access to but rarely visited.

What matters to me has changed. When it first happened there was just this sense of disbelief, and horrible pain that nobody could control. I became suicidal. I felt like I was separated from the rest of the world by a thick glass. I could see what people were doing and I could hear them, but it made no sense. I couldn't relate. I thought I was going to die. When I didn't think I was going to die, I wanted to die. I couldn't get any relief.

Over the next year and a half, what was important was just trying to hang on to the shreds of my life. I went from thinking of myself as a pretty healthy person and then finally identifying with the fact that I was this chronically sick, screwed-up, compromised individual. It got to be eighteen months and I just said, "I have to stop pretending that I'm just going to be sick for a few days and then be all right. This is my life now." I was just anguished. I cried for a month. I felt as if I was being permanently separated from the rest of the human race. I was afraid that I would become this thing kept in a back room of somebody's house. So, I developed this rationale for remaining alive, which was that even if I could do nothing, even if I was just a thing in the back room taking pain meds all the time, I would be able to have my kids come in and sit on my bed and talk to me. I could listen to them. That was it. I decided that as long as I had that, I had some reason to not kill myself.

In 2009 there was a street fair on my mother's birthday. I tried to get up and take a walk in town and I couldn't do it. I just couldn't do it. At that point it wasn't the pain—I had this sensation of weakness. I felt like my arms couldn't support anything in them, and my legs couldn't support my body.

This was not a maintainable lifestyle. I had to find someone who could help me. Once I finally found my doctor, within a month they came up with an approach and a series of antibiotics and other medications that dealt with the pain. I still felt horrible, but I could tell that there was a change. The pain became manageable.

I was actually okay as long as I took my pills. I would walk around with my pills clutched to my chest, because if I missed a dose I would be in deep trouble. I could definitely see that I was getting better. I finally did get adjusted to saying, "This is my life." I had to learn to live sick and to tell myself, "You are not a well person. You are a compromised person, and you have to find a way to do everything while you are feeling sick." I was managing.

The following November I had a relapse. I had anxiety that was so bad I couldn't get out of my bed. I was cowering in a corner. It was depersonalization. I had never felt anything like it. During that period, going to school, dragging myself to work, most of the time I had 60 percent of a life. The missing 40 percent were relationships.

I was living with this guy who was essentially taking care of me like I was a six-month-old infant. We had no quality of relationship. I didn't talk to friends. I was just angry, resentful, jealous that I couldn't do what they did. I just cut contact with them. I couldn't do it. For three years my favorite time has often been night. When I can take my pills, I can take my sleep medication and just kiss it all goodbye.

I've gotten a lot better, but with Lyme, it's not like you're sick or you're better. It's this path that you crawl up. I've been off antibiotics since March, I had been on them for almost three years, and I think by now I'm starting to trust that it's going to get better. There are people who are completely debilitated by their psychiatric symptoms, and I've always been terrified I'm going to get there, but it just hasn't happened yet.

See, people don't understand. They don't want to look at sick people. Last spring was the first time anyone in the administration at my school even noticed that I had been missing a lot of time. When they called me out, it felt like they had taken this incredible struggle that I had to survive, and were using it as a club to beat me up with. I wanted to say to them, "You don't even know what I didn't do. You didn't even notice that for two years I didn't teach a class!" It was unbelievable. I always used to talk to people about how I was feeling. Once that happened I stopped. I realized that this disease could be used to hurt you. Now, when people ask me how I'm feeling, I say "Fine." At this point, if I were contagious with typhus I would come in.

People either think you're crazy or neurotic. They think you're making it up. I have a sister who is very close to me. She is a nurse practitioner, so she is very embedded in mainstream medical care. I think at the beginning she also shared a lot of the skepticism about whether or not you're actually sick. She now works down in Raleigh, by the vet school at North Carolina State. That school is where they were doing all the *Bartonella* testing, so she heard all of the research that was being described. Doctors won't tell you about persistent Lyme, but veterinarians will. They have animals that are presenting with long-term symptoms, and animals aren't neurotic or crazy. She also saw me get sick once, and it shocked her. It just shocked her. She said I got blue in the face because I was so breathless. Now, when she talks to other people about Lyme, she says, "I saw what my sister went though. I saw her and I know her. I know what kind of healthy individual she was before this happened to her."

People don't understand this unless they've experienced it. For example, I didn't ever call what I was feeling "pain." I would tell people I had this sensation of things crawling under my skin, or I feel like I'm strung out on an electrical grid, and I can feel an electrical current running through my back. I couldn't take my focus away from it. I couldn't get away from it. It's absolutely intolerable. When I said this to my doctor he looked up at me and said, "That's pain." I had two natural childbirths, no analgesics at all. Nothing. This was more than pain. People don't understand, they just don't. Even if they think they can understand, they think, "Well what's so bad about that? Okay, you feel like your skin is crawling." You can't capture the hideous feeling that you have in words people will understand.

I was doing a lot of Buddhist meditation before I got sick, but I hadn't done enough of it. I wasn't able to deal with the pain the way you're supposed to deal with the pain. Though I loved the philosophy, I never really understood the whole empathy thing. I would read about these people who felt the suffering of the entire world and wanted to take it away, and I just I didn't get that. At one point after I got sick, I was on a trip in Paris. We were in a restaurant and there was this old woman who was waiting on us. You could tell she didn't like Americans; she didn't like tourists. She was really crotchety. During the meal she said something really rude to one of my nieces and I remember thinking, "Oh my God, I wonder if she's in pain." I said, "I bet that she's in pain." I realized then, it was the first time in my life really, that I understood what she was feeling. This experience has actually made me sort of empathetic for the first time in my life. I was fifty-eight years old. I will never be one of those people who say, "I'm glad it happened." I'm not, I feel like it's robbed me of a lot, but it has made me a deeper person.

There are so many people out there who don't get what I got. They don't find the amazing Lyme guy, and they just live these horrible, horrible lives. I know a woman who was on IV for three and a half years. She had a total vascular collapse and had a headache for six years. She almost died a few times. Finally she found this alternative treatment that helped her. I mean, within a year she was functioning again. This woman had no cognitive function. She couldn't remember her name. I can't help but think about all the people who are like her, who don't find that treatment. If you go to Bear Mountain Park in the summer, you can see all these people from the city sitting on the grass by the lake. Every time I see them I want to scream, "Get off the grass!" There just have to be people in that population who go back to New York and get sick, and then what do they do?

Not enough people know. Well, they think they know, but they label you as neurotic, or as a malingerer. People need to know. I find that I can't ever forget this, even when I would like to. It changes you. It's not something you can opt out of. You can't say, "I'm not going to be like that." It just doesn't work. Your perceptions are altered. Your brain chemistry is altered in a way that makes you not human.

That's what I want to say: It makes you not human.

CHAPTER 11

DR. EDWARD ZORIN

Dr. Zorin, fifty-eight, was the first person I met who seemed reluctant to share his story. We met outside the New York Public Library. When I saw him navigating his way up the grand steps, his face was focused on his Blackberry and showed no signs of pain. When we saw each other, I recognized an urgency and fear in his eyes, the kind that you do not want to get in the way of. His thick New York accent broke the air when he spoke, and he shook my hand with a firmness I did not expect from a fellow Lyme patient.

Lyme physicians who come to know personally the struggles for treatment, diagnosis, and acceptance patients experience often choose to break away from the mainstream medical system to open their own practices. I expected this might be the case with Dr. Zorin, so I was surprised by his pushback against this idea. Though I understood his resistance, I was also saddened that many of us with both the knowledge and the means to help people living with this disease are too scared to do so. The fear of discussion that surrounds chronic Lyme was palpable during my interview with Edward Zorin.

The following is composed from my notes on our meeting that day.

We can just do this out here, can't we? I've got to get back to work pretty quick. I don't need any of your emotional bullshit, and I will sign whatever you want me to sign, but I don't want to be recorded. Professional reasons, okay? Good. I'm going to give it to you straight.

In 2009, I had a private practice where I worked as an internist seeing primarily older people for their regular checkups. My schedule was normally pretty full, but I always made sure to take some time for a walk in the park during lunch—helps me process the day, you know? I don't know the day, never saw a bug or a ring, but I'm convinced I must have contracted Lyme disease during one of my treks across the park. It was probably during one of the days when my socks didn't come up high enough on my ankles. Sometimes that happens.

So honestly, during my entire medical career up until that point, I had called in sick five times. I was always a healthy guy and really did not like to miss work, but one day I woke up with Bell's palsy on the left side of my face, paralysis in my neck, and blurred vision. I knew I needed to stay home. As a physician, I had seen cases of Lyme before. I knew the early warning signs and the symptoms of late-stage Lyme, but I never had understood the pain that my patients described until I tried to move my neck that morning. I started to scream. After three days of this pain and paralysis, I decided that I must have been showing symptoms of advanced Lyme, thinking that any previous symptoms had gone unnoticed. It wasn't hard to believe. I'm a doctor with a busy schedule; headaches, fatigue, and joint pain can easily be explained away as stress or the result of lack of sleep. Plus, I was almost forty. I was starting to get old.

I knew how unreliable blood tests could be, so I didn't even bother messing with them. I called a friend who went to medical school with me and asked to be treated for Lyme with three months of IV Rocephin. I knew it wasn't exactly by the book, but I got lucky. My buddy trusted my judgment and wrote me a prescription. To avoid letting anyone at work know I had Lyme, I arranged treatment at a walk-in clinic. A different nurse or a different doctor treated me every day, and many of them had never even heard of Lyme being treated intravenously. But even when I was at my sickest, I like to think my presence was commanding enough that none of the nurses or doctors were going to mess with me.

Within only one month of aggressive treatment, I was back on my feet and back at work. I felt healthy again. The treatment was obviously no easy trip, but as I worked through it I could feel my body fighting the war against those spirochete bitches swimming around in my blood.

It was only after I finished the treatment, and only after I was back at work, that I asked for the Western blot blood test. Unfortunately, it came back positive, but I wasn't going to let a positive blood test ruin my life, you know? I just had to accept that I was going to have to keep on fighting a battle against these assholes. If I stayed on the offensive, I knew I would be okay. Now, I just take a course of antibiotics every spring. Around then I can always feel my body bitching out. Who knows, maybe it's cyclical or something. So I take some drugs in the spring, four weeks normally, and that's that. You know what? I've never felt better.

I know there are a bunch of Lyme specialists out there who got their start because they were patients of this themselves. But I have to be honest with you—I have never considered treating Lyme patients since I got sick. I don't want to have to deal with all that political bullshit. Whenever I see a patient with what looks like Lyme I immediately refer them to a Lyme-literate doctor, but I just don't want to risk treating it myself. The other problem is that many of my patients are older, and they don't notice their symptoms are abnormal until it's too late.

Look, this isn't going to kill anyone if they know what is happening in their body and they treat it aggressively enough. You have to pull out the big guns with Lyme as soon as possible. If you do, you'll turn out like me. If you don't—well I'm sorry for the people who don't.

So, good. You have everything you need? Nice to meet you. Got to get back to work.

INTERLUDE

With the exception of Dr. Zorin, everyone I spoke to was surprisingly willing to share their story. I was impressed by this, and at times was embarrassed by my struggle to talk about my own experience. While many of the people I connected with did struggle to reflect on what had happened to them—and almost all didn't want to use their real names—they also seemed to feel empowered by the simple act of speaking their stories out loud. Like Dr. Zorin, I hadn't found that yet. I still lowered my voice when I was asked to explain my interest in chronic Lyme narratives, to explain just how and why I got involved.

CHAPTER 12

ELLA MCGOVERN

On the phone Ella McGovern, forty-five, was cheerful, a tone matched by the ambiance of her home, which was airy and light—not the setting you'd expect for some of the hardship and pain she described. Her story crystalized for me something I had up until then not fully realized: many chronic Lyme patients who lack support, both emotional and medical, will struggle with even the most basic, routine activities. Going to the bathroom, getting up the stairs, preparing meals: these things can't be done alone. How can we expect people to heal when so many are left without anyone to help them? While thankfully Ella has had familial support, her struggle made the absolute necessity of that type of support impossible to ignore.

I was first diagnosed in 1992, so it's been quite a while for me. They didn't originally know what I had. They said it was MS, then ALS, then conversion disorder, and then finally Lyme. I was hospitalized and in a wheelchair and [for the longest time] they had no solid diagnosis for me. Scary stuff.

It began with pure exhaustion. At the time I was working in New York City for an investment bank and was used to working ten- or twelve-hour days. I was going back to school for my MBA and getting a Series 7 license, so I was used to pulling crazy hours, but I got to a place where I just couldn't keep up with it. I hid it at work for a while. I did all these little things, like laughing and making little to-do lists and hiding notes here and there, but then one day I walked in and I didn't know where my desk was. I didn't recognize the floor I worked on. It was just dangerous. So I had to go out on disability; there was no other choice. I put myself right into therapy, but just wasn't getting anywhere. I didn't know what to do. The therapist was sending me to a neurologist, and the neurologist would send me back to the therapist. I got a little better and tried to go back to work, but then all these physical symptoms started to come into play.

I would get migraines every three days or so. They would hit and I would be out for at least five hours, curled up on the floor in a back office with a migraine. I mean, come on, you can't do that. Then I started to notice I was losing strength in my legs. I realized I was having trouble stepping up onto the bus. Then I was dragging myself up those steps. I couldn't walk to the back of the bus. It was just getting progressively worse. One day I was walking from my office to the bus stop, and it was raining. The benches were all taken, and I was wearing this light colored suit that I loved, it was so expensive. I got so tired that I couldn't walk anymore and had to sit down on the ground. I totally wrecked my suit, but I had no other choice. Meanwhile the doctors were telling me nothing was wrong. So, I thought nothing was wrong. I just thought I needed to keep pushing forward.

I did see one infectious disease doctor very early on who told me go to on IV for the Lyme. My primary care doctor really thought that something was wrong, knew something was wrong. He wasn't 100 percent confident that it was Lyme but wanted me to try the treatment. I said I'd do it, but when the insurance company denied it the opportunity just slipped away. Eventually I wasn't pulling my own weight at work. I could tell that if I didn't go out on disability sooner rather than later, they were going to start to penalize me for not doing my job. Because I wasn't doing my job: I was asking people to help me with the stuff I wasn't physically able to do.

My mom had Lyme disease and had seen a Lyme doctor who was a psychiatrist as well as a Lyme specialist, so we thought he might be able to look at the whole case. I didn't care if it was psychological or if it was Lyme, I just wanted to start moving forward with some sort of treatment. I wanted to start walking again—anything, really, would have been nice. He looked at everything and said, absolutely, this is Lyme, and he got me on IV right away. Within two weeks I saw improvement. It wasn't a miracle cure. I wasn't up walking or anything, but I think I could crawl a little bit when I went to him. It was a lot of improvement. But insurance changed, and I had to go to another Lyme doctor. I finally got strong enough to go to an inpatient rehabilitation hospital. I planned on coming out of there walking; [instead] I came out with a better wheelchair. I was able to be a lot more independent and actually moved [back] out of my parent's house and into here. That was in 1996. My parent's house wasn't handicap accessible, so I had to crawl to a lot of rooms and stuff.

About every five years I feel like I relapse. During my first relapse my doctor's insurance changed, and I was forced to change doctors again. That's when I found my current doctor. I didn't even realize he was here, fifteen minutes from my backyard. He was the first person who looked into the co-infections. And, lo and behold, that's where the *Babesia* popped up. Once I was treated for *Babesia*, a lot changed. I stopped having night sweats, which before I never had even counted as a symptom. I just had to change my sheets and pajamas in the middle of the night, but that didn't even register as something bad compared to everything else. I also started to get some sensation back in my legs and eventually started to walk again. It was a miracle.

Over two years, I had to teach myself how to walk again. I had to say to myself, "Pick up your leg and take a step." Now I couldn't even explain it to you because it's so natural, but I remember when I was trying to do it again, I had to try to think about activating specific muscles to move my leg. When you are in a wheelchair, they tell you to try and move your legs whenever you made a weight transfer. I always told my legs to push, but they just never did anything. I started feeling something in my legs again once I did the *Babesia* treatment. It was like things started sparking. I told my legs to push and they did, but they started going crazy. I flipped myself over in the wheelchair a couple times, but my legs were moving! Obviously there was some connection that was going through that wasn't going through before. Those were some exciting falls. And now I can walk, I can do a tiny bit of a run, and even a little jump. Jumping is hard. There are a lot of muscles involved in a tiny little jump, you wouldn't believe it. There are definitely still some limitations, but compared to where I was, I don't even like to think about that.

Today, my symptoms aren't gone, but they are definitely at bay. The last six months have been really nice. I've been able to go out a little bit more. I can go to the grocery store and do some shopping. It depends on how loud the loudspeakers are and stuff like that, but that's good for me. I've gone out a couple times with my parents for dinner and stuff. It's nice to be able to go out and feel like I'm part of the world again. You don't realize how shut-in you are when you can't go out to anyplace public.

I don't like to give percentages; it's so hard to think of how long it's been since I was 100 percent. All I can think of is 100 percent of what, of which me? Am I really thrilled with where I'm at right now? Yeah! Because it's better than where I was a year ago. Are there still a lot of things I want to have better? Yeah. I want to go back to work. I want to be an active member of society. But I'll take what I have because it's still a lot better than where I was.

I think that people who have experienced true sickness understand a certain language. Someone who knows pain will understand. I've talked to other neighbors who don't have Lyme but who have MS or cancer, and they get it. When you say I'm just so tired today, or this is not a good day, they understand what that means. A normal person who hasn't been sick, who hasn't dealt with real pain or real hurt, is going to think that getting their hand caught in a drawer really hurts. To them, it does. So they can't appreciate other kinds of pain. Just last week, I was so dizzy I had to sleep on the bathroom floor. I keep towels and a little pillow there because that happens to me all the time. People don't get that. Who would even think of that? I don't blame them for not understanding. I just want people to acknowledge that things are different for me; I'm working in a different set of parameters.

What I don't understand is why Lyme is being thrown under the carpet as not existing, hard to catch, easy to cure in twenty days. That needs to change. I want to promote the concept of looking at this economically. Look at my case: if I had gotten treated with that IV antibiotic within the first year of my infection, think of all the money that probably could have been saved. The CDC and the NIH are actively promoting the IDSA guidelines. Why are government agencies backing treatment guidelines that allow so many patients to wind up with chronic debilitating symptoms because of insufficient treatment? At least 300,000 people per year get Lyme, and about 15 percent of those people have remaining symptoms. This works out to about a $4.5-billion cost to society for chronic Lyme over the last ten years. I would think federal agencies would be backing guidelines that would lower that cost.

So, 300,000 times 15 percent equals 45,000. That's 45,000 people with remaining Lyme symptoms per year, and 450,000 people with remaining symptoms in the last ten years. If you attribute $10,000 per person of government spending on disability checks, loss of work, medical expenses, and the like, then $4,500,000,000 have been wasted on chronic Lyme disease in the last decade. Why aren't we considering offering people more than thirty days of oral antibiotics to see if they can become symptom-free in the beginning?

Even if we accept that they don't want to approve IV treatment, why wouldn't they extend the oral treatment time? Why not two months of Doxy? It's not expensive. People take Doxy for years for acne and have no trouble getting approved for treatment. It doesn't make financial sense on any level. If it were just the insurance companies, or if someone was making money, I would understand. No one is making money on this. No one is saving face. So what is it? What's going on? The math doesn't work out. It's as simple as that. Something bigger is happening behind the scenes with this disease. I know it.

CHAPTER 13

DAVE RITEMAN

Dave Riteman, twenty-two, grew up just minutes from Bard College. We met during one of my visits to the local support group. I remember he sat next to his mom during the meeting and didn't speak much throughout; she did most of the talking. On my way out, she asked if I'd like to grab a cup of coffee with her son.

The following are excerpts from his interview transcript.

None of my friends know. They all think I changed schools because I wasn't doing well in my old school. I guess in a way they were right. At first I didn't tell them because I didn't know how they would react. I didn't want a pity party, you know? But then I told this kid, Bill. He used to be my best friend. We played Little League together in elementary school and stayed super-close forever. But when I told him what was going on he got so weird. It was like he was grossed out or freaked out or something. He'd do weird stuff, like change his seat in science class or stop coming over to my house. So after a while that friendship kind of died out. Which is sad, you know? I'm not an alien or anything. I just have Lyme disease.

At first, I didn't think it had anything to do with Lyme. I just thought sick people grossed him out. Which I got—I mean I think sick people gross me out too. I go get IV at this clinic and always try to avoid making eye contact with all the cancer people. I know I can't catch it or anything, but I don't know, there is just something scary about that. Death isn't something people want to face. But I'm not dying; my body is just like buggin' out . . . Anyway, this kid Bill's mom eventually called my mom and told her that Bill was feeling uncomfortable hanging out with me because he thought I had a mental disorder. So yeah. That sucked, but that was that.

I just don't tell people about this anymore. I'm not going to walk around explaining what it means to have serious Lyme disease, if people are just going to think I'm a crazy person no matter what I say. I'm just not going to. It feels like losing, over and over again. I'm normally pretty good at keeping the pain all under wraps and I've been really lucky to not have any neurological issues yet. I can still talk fine and remember things and everything, so that's definitely good. What it is, mostly, for me is muscle pain. It's sort of like after a big workout, you know? Moving around you have really achy legs, or arms, or abs, or whatever. It's a similar feeling but they don't ache, they burn. They feel so tired all the time that any movement, like even reaching for your cell phone, sets them on fire. Yeah, that's what it is. It's like fire under your skin. You can always sort of feel it there if you don't move around, but even the littlest movements—like talking to you right now—turns up the heat. Can you imagine that? Maybe you can. But most people can't. They say, "Oh yeah, your muscles feel like they are on fire. Right." But they can't get past feeling shitty after a workout. It's so much more than that. No one gets it.

I used to play for my high school soccer team. Girls liked me, boys liked me; everyone did. Once I got sick, my life became this horrible cocktail of me feeling like I couldn't connect with people and people not wanting to connect with me. Ultimately, at the end of tenth grade I had to change schools. It was for a couple of reasons: we wanted to move to New York to be closer to better doctors, my parents got divorced, I wasn't doing well in my classes, and I was convinced that everyone hated me. I wonder sometimes how much of that was in my head. Because I've gotten a lot better over the last two years. I can really feel the difference in the way I interact with people. I'm so much less angry, and my temper has really calmed down. So that's helped me make some new friends, who I know now not to tell about Lyme. There are still some things that just won't go away. But Bill's mom, she was a doctor in Maryland where I used to live— she said that I was probably going to experience psychosomatic pain for a while until I dealt with my psychological problems.

Here's the thing about that though. I do deal with my psychological problems. People say I'm depressed. Of course I'm fucking depressed! I wake up every morning and my arms are on fire, I had to quit my soccer team, I lost all of my friends, my dad left, I have to take tons of drugs every day, no girl has kissed me since I was fifteen. If I weren't depressed, there would be something seriously wrong with me. I deal with that. My mom takes me to a therapist three times a week. Just because I'm not medicated doesn't mean I'm not dealing with it. See, I wish I was just depressed, or had bipolar disorder or some shit, because then I could go on some medicine and start to get normal again, or at least closer to normal. Where I am right now is that I take medicine for six months, I feel better—normal— and then six months later I'm back to where I started. Seriously, depression sounds easier than this.

I know I sound angry, and I'm sorry if that's not what you wanted from me, but I'd be lying to you if I didn't tell you how angry I am. I didn't get to have the high school experience everyone else got to have. I didn't go away to college, and once I thought I was going to get recruited to play soccer. Now I'm taking classes at the local community college because I don't want to move to far away from my doctor, and I can't afford much else because of the medical bills. It's already put such a strain on my mom, I can't ask much more from her. So yes, I'm angry. I want insurance to help my mom pay to keep me healthy. I want people to start doing more research about how they can help me, or get rid of these ticks, or find an actual cure, or something. I want something more than I have. This life is not the life I wanted. It's just not.

I told you before that I'm not dying, but I sort of wish I was. I'm not going to kill myself or anything, but sometimes that feels like the only way out. Did you ever think about that? I have enough pills in my medicine cabinet to do it. I probably could. Don't worry. I won't. I want to get better too badly to do that. But it's tempting sometimes. It seems like it might be the right way out.

I hope me telling you all this has been helpful. I don't talk about it too much with people my age, so I think it's probably good for me. My therapist will be happy. Look, just do me a favor and make people want to change this. This isn't cancer; it shouldn't be impossible to cure. So let's find something that will do it. Let's get people excited about making this go away. Maybe then I'll get my life back. I haven't given up hope yet. Seriously, I know it might sound like that but I promise you, I haven't given up hope yet.

CHAPTER 14

LAURA WILLIAMS

Though the region I call home reports the highest rates of Lyme infection in the world, Lyme disease is not limited to the American Northeast, where most of my interviewees contracted their disease. As Lyme disease is a global phenomenon, in order to get a better understanding of the global chronic Lyme experience, I'd need to connect with fellow sufferers well beyond my horizons.

Laura Williams, forty-four, lives in Australia. The following is composed of excerpts from our interview via Skype.

This is my story. In 1987 I was bitten by a tick in Japan and was very sick for many, many years. I was finally diagnosed with Lyme disease in 2005. I spent eight years in a wheelchair unable to wash, dress, or feed myself. Unfortunately, I had transmitted the disease to my twin girls before they were born. They are now eighteen and have been sick their entire lives.

When I was first diagnosed I didn't know anyone else with Lyme disease. I had never even heard the words "Lyme disease." It's not actually as rare as the government would like to admit, but according to our health organizations, we don't have Lyme disease in Australia. There are actually a lot of people that have it, but many undiagnosed people. So there is very little support for people the whole time. When I was first diagnosed, there were only two groups that helped support patients of Lyme disease. There was one support network in Sydney called TAGS: the Tick Advisory Group of Sydney, and died out in the early 2000s, so a Yahoo email group was the only resource for Australian Lyme patients in 2005. [TAGS is now Tick Alert Group Support.[44]] That was only thirteen years ago. I joined that, and I found a specialist in Sydney who helped me get the Lyme diagnosis but wouldn't treat me. So I originally was treated by my GP, who knew as little about Lyme as I did. We relied on the support of this email group in the earliest stages of my treatment, and also spent a lot of time connecting with U.S.-based Lyme disease experts by phone. I just wasn't getting better, and eventually we realized I needed to go to America to get the treatment I really needed. When we got there, American doctors saved my life. I had a dramatic improvement. Back at home my GP, who I love, and I had been working on treatment but we really didn't know what we were doing. I needed people who knew enough to help turn my life around.

While I was living in America and receiving my treatment, the Lyme community in Australia started to explode. More people started to join the email list, and a lot of conversation started up about changing the way Lyme was viewed in Australia. In response to this stir and new interest, the Lyme Disease Association of Australia was started, and I actually took over as president of the LDAA in 2010. Once I took over the Lyme Disease Association, the group became significantly more active. We're working to provide services and information to everyone who asks for it, and that number continues to grow. We have over a thousand people contacting the LDAA every year. I probably do forty hours a week with the LDAA. I'd like to get paid. That would be nice. But I do it because I love it, and I want to help people as much as possible.

We're also not only focused on patient advocacy any more, we hope to change the treatment and diagnosis process of Lyme in our country.

The Lyme strain we have in Australia is more similar to MS, Parkinson's, or ALS, whereas the classic Lyme in America is more focused on joints. I know that you have a lot of neurological issues now, it's kind of changing, but we've been dealing with that from the start. The Australian strain is very hard to diagnose and difficult to treat. There is no test for the Australian strain of Lyme disease right now, but research into finding the Australian strain of Lyme disease is slowly progressing.

It's all a slow process though. There are currently fifty doctors treating around 200,000 Lyme disease patients in this country. For a long time, we were forced to recommended that people go overseas for treatment because no one can, or will, help patients anywhere close to home. But that is slowly changing as more doctors become Lyme-aware and train specifically in Lyme disease treatment. I created this doctor's information kit with the LDAA, so that local doctors can help Lyme patients without being completely in the dark, but a lot of doctors still refuse to even take it.

The Australian healthcare system is universal. So, everyone in Australia is guaranteed healthcare, almost all of which is paid for by the government. The health department of New South Wales, our largest population state, dictates most of the policy that ultimately covers the rest of the country. When it comes to treating infectious disease, and getting insurance for that treatment, doctors need to rely on government standards, and can only treat diseases that the health department publicly acknowledges are present in the country. If the health department does not list a disease on their site, doctors find it difficult to treat. Lyme disease is not listed as an infectious disease in Australia, so our medical professionals risk getting penalized for treating the disease, even if patients are infected overseas.

We're waiting for that to change. A couple of weeks ago we actually staged a protest in Sydney, and that had one hundred and fifty people in it. See, there have been four studies done in Australia about Lyme disease, about whether it's here. One of them didn't find Lyme, three of them did.

The health department of New South Wales looked at the negative study and decided that there was no Lyme disease in Australia. People should be able to get treatment, and doctors should be able to provide that treatment without being penalized for doing that. We brought those demands to the government, but getting them there wasn't the easiest thing.

You'll get a kick out of this. I actually had to do some sneaky, behind-the-scenes stuff. About a year ago I sent in a Freedom of Information request asking how New South Wales Health [Department] wrote their Lyme disease policy. I've been sending these requests for twelve months now, and they keep losing my application. So at our protest, instead of posting it we actually hand-delivered it. They wouldn't let me in the door of the building, so we sent a young woman in a very short skirt up the stairs and she literally put the request in the security guard's hand. It actually got to the right department! Now that they accepted the request, the LDAA will be able to see what evidence was excluded in the decision not to include Lyme on the list of infectious diseases present in the country. I know that in 2011, when they updated the policy, there were no current Lyme researchers or patient advocates on the panel, which probably enabled them to ignore information that would have proved the presence of Lyme here in Australia. Once we have that information, we can start our negotiations about trying to get a proper policy in place.

What struck me most about the protest was that Lyme had negatively affected all of the individuals gathered there that day. People were holding up posters saying, MY MOMMY HAS LYME DISEASE. There were little girls in wheelchairs, and whole families that were dramatically impacted. It has just ruined so many people's lives. I find that so sad. It's so unnecessary that so many lives have been impacted. It was really overwhelming.

At one point, I was standing at the back of the crowd, speaking to a woman who was very upset. When I turned around to walk back towards the front of the protest, a stream of people were waiting to speak to me as well. They were coming up to me and grabbing my hand and holding it and looking in my eyes and saying, "You saved me." I felt sort of like a politician in the mall shaking everyone's hands. I was going down the line shaking hands and having people thank me for the smallest things, with such gratitude in their eyes. They came to meet me and said, "Thank you, you've saved my life." Other people did that for me. I see it as paying it forward.

As powerful as it was, there was something really disturbing about it to me. I should not have been the person these individuals went to speak to. They should be able to speak to their doctors, or specialists, about their infectious disease. I should not know more than doctors about this disease.

Lyme disease turns seemingly intelligent people mute. I truly, truly don't understand it: why they have prevented research and treatment for this disease over and over again. One of the reasons is that the people who wrote the one study that didn't find Lyme disease then went on to make a name for themselves. They went everywhere. They told whoever would listen that Lyme disease didn't exist in Australia. They are famous, but they don't listen to reason.

Now though, the number of people on our side is growing. There's a large group of people on the forums, and on the email lists, and on Yahoo, and Facebook, who are constantly supporting each other, and together they are starting to drive the political conversation. Two of the four public television stations have run programs on Lyme in the last few months. It's becoming a lot more mainstream. For example, there is a group in Australia called the CWA, the Country Women's Association, and they've decided to make Lyme disease their pick project for next year. The last thing you want to do is really annoy the CWA. They really get cranky. They are these little old ladies in curls with gray and purple hair making cakes and pushing for progress on issues they care about. We had huge droughts in Australia for ten or fifteen years, and they pushed for not only assistance but also financial assistance, and counseling for a lot of the farmers to help stop the high suicide rate. Once they pick an issue, they wear government into the ground. A couple of their members are attempting to get the main body to pick Lyme and I think it may happen. We'll see.

There is hype here, I think anyway, because it hasn't been recognized in Australia as a disease. My doctor had never even heard of Lyme disease when I was diagnosed in 2005. Whereas now, if I'm wearing my LDAA T-shirt, people will stop me and say, "Oh I've heard of Lyme disease." But still, when people say, "I think I've got Lyme disease" and the person says, "Oh no you can't have Lyme disease. There's no Lyme in Australia," it makes it very difficult for the word to spread. We need to keep talking about it.

Luckily I'm pretty good at talking! And I still want to put my time and focus on Lyme because one of my daughters is still very sick. We still hope she can completely recover, but it's hard to say. I mean, I spent eight years in an electric wheelchair unable to wash, dress, or feed myself. My husband had to cut up all my food for me. And I'm pretty much back to normal. So we'll just see about my baby girl.

When I first got sick. I started off with a kind of chronic fatigue problem, which then led to digestive problems. They were so bad that I lost twenty-six kilos [fifty-seven pounds] in twelve months. I had constant diarrhea. After the digestive problems, my neurological problems started. I started having trouble walking and at times problems talking. I had all the brain fog and all the cognitive stuff that I didn't even know was there until it went away. It's like the frog in a beaker, you know? If you put a frog in boiling water it jumps out, but if you put it in cold water and slowly heat it, the frog will boil to death. I was like that. My symptoms happened slowly over time, so I put up with them for a long time.

I was gradually getting sicker and sicker. I was misdiagnosed a number of times with lupus, fibromyalgia, chronic fatigue, none of which are treated with the antibiotics I needed. Ultimately, I was confined to my bed or wheelchair. Leaving the house required an almost impossible effort. My general practitioner was convinced that I was suffering from ALS, and I agreed I would get tested, but only once I had ruled everything else out. My doctor gave me his log-in password for all of the medical databases so that I could do whatever research I felt was necessary to get on board with his diagnosis. When I found Lyme disease, I instantly knew that was what I had. I had the most classic case: I was bitten, I remember the tick bite, and my friend squeezed it as she pulled it out, I got the rash, and I got the flu afterwards. It was classic.

When I showed the description of the disease to my doctor, he said, "I don't know anything about this. You do the research, you tell me what you want me to treat you with, and I'll do it." There was really only one doctor in Australia treating Lyme at the time, so I traveled to Sydney to see this professor, who has since decided that it's too controversial and no longer treats Lyme patients. He diagnosed me but refused to treat, so I got the treatment guidelines from ILADS in the U.S., and started working on those with my GP. It definitely helped. It stopped me dying—I was having organs shut down and all sorts of things—but it wasn't enough. That year, my grandmother very sadly died, but she left me some money, and that's how I was able to go to America to get treatment. My GP has really been fantastic. The times that we have had problems he's really gone up to bat for us.

The reality of the situation is that infectious disease doctors in my country do not believe in Lyme disease. The fact that my family and I found a doctor who was able and willing to accept the possibility of Lyme was incredibly lucky. When my daughter was very sick, doctors in the local hospital actively tried to stop her from getting treatment. She was completely paralyzed, struggling to breathe, and the hospital threatened to turn her away. I mean, she was obviously faking, right? My daughter was lying on the table between the hospital doctor and me, and I was forced to call my GP on his cell phone to try and convince the specialist to treat my child. Even after speaking to another medical practitioner, the hospital still refused to treat my daughter. The nurses handed her back to us and said, "When she stops breathing, bring her back."

I feel guilty sometimes. I spent about a third of my pregnancy in the hospital because I was so sick, and we didn't know the girls would be sick with Lyme when they were first born. I have twin girls. One of my girls has been sick since she was born. She went on to develop epilepsy, ADD, Asperger's, and severe dyslexia. Later in her life, she was bitten by a tick and infected when we were on vacation. By the time we got back to Australia her body just couldn't cope. Within about twelve months of her infection, she was in a wheelchair.

We're turning a corner now though. We all are. We'll get the government's support now and more people's lives will be fixed early. My goal is in ten years' time, I'll be healthy, my girls will be healthy, and it will be unusual to have Lyme disease for fifteen years before you're diagnosed. We want to catch it early. We want to get better. It's has to get done.

INTERLUDE

My interviews took on a very different tone once I met with Laura. Though I was still incredibly moved by the bravery and strength of the individuals I spoke with, I no longer left our meetings with a sense of awe, wonder, or sadness. Instead, I realized that these stories could do a lot more than simply validate my own experience. Together, they communicated the voice of a population that had been silenced by medical and social prejudice and ignorance. From this point forward, I left my interviews with a sense of purpose, a new sense of agenda.

CHAPTER 15

CHARLIE CRAWFORD

Originally from the suburbs of New York City, Charlie Crawford, fifty-seven, lives and works in Singapore, where Lyme disease is virtually unknown. Doctors do not learn about it in medical school, as it is not believed to be present in the country. In reality, however, Lyme is regularly diagnosed around the world, and bacterial strains of tick-borne diseases often differ depending on where the disease is contracted in the world. Charlie is currently traveling from Singapore back to the United States in search of treatment for his worsening condition, which most of his doctors at home have never even heard of.

While it's easy to worry about the state of the American medical system and its treatment of Lyme, it's just as easy to forget that Lyme patients here may be lucky to have 50 percent of doctors rallying behind the chronic Lyme cry. Elsewhere, the vast majority of doctors have never even heard of the disease.

The following is a compilation from my email exchanges with Charlie.

As Lyme is considered a Northern Hemisphere ailment, it's almost unknown here in Singapore. I was only lucky that my doctor had a patient who recently returned from Norway and had just been infected. He caught it early and was treated with the normal month-long antibiotic "cure." It's only because of that experience that my doctor even thought to test for Lyme. Over the course of the past year I've been speaking with him about what seems to be called chronic Lyme disease.

I think I must have been infected in November of 2007, when I was at home in Redding, Connecticut, with my parents. I was there for about a week, packing up all of my possessions that had languished in my parents' basement since I moved to Asia in 1988. I noticed my first symptoms appear in April of 2008 when I began to have knee problems. My doctor thought I must have arthritis, and eventually talked of an immune suppressant disorder, but things came and went, and with painkillers I was able to push through until things seemed to go back to normal.

Throughout 2009 I had occasional joint inflammations, but even when the medics extracted fluid, they could only determine that my white blood cell count was inordinately high. My doctor still had no clue as to what was going wrong. It was unnerving. In 2010 I took a year's sabbatical from work, and when I was traveling around the world, I faced a series of flu-like ailments. I could only describe this as constant fatigue. I also had these horrible night sweats that forced me to change my clothes in the middle of the night. At this point I was still unaware of what was happening to me.

Months later I had a night where I had this incredible pain in my hip. I stayed awake the entire night crying, unable to find a tolerable position to rest in. I eventually had to take myself to the hospital, but again they had no answers for me. Though he was unsure of the cause, my doctor recommended we undergo a weekend of antibiotic drips. I didn't understand what it was meant to treat; all I knew was that the nurses were all amazed at the strength of the treatment I was prescribed. It was on this occasion that my doctor tested for Lyme and it came back positive. He put me on one month of oral antibiotics, suggesting that I would now be cured. But I'm not, not at all.

My toes and feet have been becoming more and more numb. At first my doctor thought it was diabetes. Eventually he referred me to a neurologist who confirmed that I have inhibited nerve function in my legs. Since that diagnosis I have had countless blood tests, brain scans, and PET scans; all to find the "cause" of my nerve damage; and all to no avail. They can't find anything wrong with me. I am the healthiest ill person my doctor has ever seen.

I'm convinced it must still be the Lyme. I've heard about the way it presents itself in people around the world, and it seems very similar to my experience. Every day it becomes harder to walk and more painful to stand. I've been traveling back and forth to America to try to find a doctor who will help tell me what is happening in my body. My life is in Singapore, yet the level of knowledge of Lyme is extremely limited. I'm trying to forge a working relationship between my Lyme doctor and my Singapore doctor. All I can do is hope and struggle forward. Nothing has worked yet.

INTERLUDE

I started feeling a sense of community with those who also intimately understand chronic Lyme. And though my interviews broadened that community to encompass countries I'd never visited—Japan, Australia, Singapore—it still felt like one unified experience. Everyone I spoke to knew of the same doctors, and had tried the same treatments. We all spoke the same language, one understood by thousands of fellow Lyme sufferers we'd never know—and yet a language we struggled to communicate to the people we do know: those who don't understand life with this disease.

CHAPTER 16

SARAH THOMAS

I met with Sarah Thomas, forty-eight, and her son James, seventeen, in their kitchen, eating biscuits made earlier that day in a middle school "home-ec" class. They lived in New Canaan, Connecticut, a town not all that different from Katonah or Bedford, wealthy suburbs of New York where life appears beautifully simple until you peek beneath the surface. As James wasn't yet eighteen, Sarah participated as well: I essentially interviewed both of them in turn. I was impressed by the ease with which Sarah spoke of her son's experience—which she did while tidying their already pristine kitchen.

The following are excerpts from her interview transcript.

I knew it wasn't normal for a second-grader to have migraines. I knew that. But I took him to doctors—it wasn't like I just sat back and let it all happen. I took him to a neurologist for the migraines. When he started having vision problems, I took him to an optometrist. He had this weird skin stuff, so I brought him to a dermatologist. Then I brought him to a rheumatologist when the muscle pain started. No one connected the dots. Everyone was treating symptoms. Symptoms, symptoms, symptoms. By the end of seventh grade he had missed fifty-five days of school. We would get in the car to go somewhere, park, hop out, and he would still be sitting there not moving. It was like having a son who acted like a ninety-year-old arthritic man. By the end of his seventh-grade year I demanded blood work. Something was terribly wrong. I knew it.

We were so lucky. He tested off-the-charts positive for Lyme. There is a sixty-forty chance that you will have a positive result even if you are infected, and I was so relieved that we were able to get a diagnosis. I took him to this Lyme specialist who immediately turned me off. He asked James what he thought they should do. Can you imagine? Asking a seventh-grader what treatment he wanted? We needed another doctor. That's when we found James's favorite doctor, our godsend. He started James on a cocktail of oral antibiotics, and it was working to some extent. He was getting out of bed, he was functioning, and he was getting himself to school. There was progress. But the antibiotics are strong, and you can't stay on them forever. The spirochetes come back, and they just get used to what's in your body. So when we would take him off for a little while, he would seriously fall back. He would get so sick.

After a few years of this our insurance dropped us. Since then, we've had to spend $100,000 on his medical care, and I just thank God that we have the money to do it. I will do anything for my child to get him better. The downside was that he still was not better! And the medicine we were paying for wasn't making him better! I think we are back up on the uptick now, though. We've started doing everything holistically. It's still very expensive, but I think it's working.

We got on the holistic route when we went to see a doctor who works very closely with these machines called Rife machines. It's very interesting, and it's all based in electricity. It ended up not being for James, but it really helped my husband to understand what was happening to our son. See, my husband is a very analytical man. Through all these years of dealing with Lyme there really wasn't anything he could scientifically see. When he sat there and watched the doctor run these electrical charges through our son, he could see on graphs and charts on the computer monitor showing where there were problems. James had every co-infection that exists with Lyme. Every one. And there they all were showing up on the computer screen. You can see it! You have this, you have this, and you have this. My husband was just blown away. He really wanted us to work with the machine, but James wasn't ready to leave his Lyme doctor yet. He trusted him.

The next thing we tried were Bicillin shots, and James hated those. They hurt him. That killed me. You know, he's had to grow up so fast because of all this, but I know he's still just a little kid. Anyway, when that didn't work, James's doctor told us he was baffled. He just threw up his hands and told us he didn't know what to try next. So, he sent us to another doctor, who really opened my mind up to the positive effects vitamins and supplements can have. A couple of months ago I found these "bio meds." They are all vitamins, powdered vitamins, and I think they are working. He is getting better. This is the first time—three and a half months of no antibiotics. We've never gone that far. He's doing great. It's just such a relief, because this has not been an easy road. Our pediatrician told us that half the medical community believes in Lyme and half doesn't. He said he was "on the fence." I'm not on the fence. He has Lyme disease. I mean, come on! We're in Connecticut. There is such a thing as Lyme in this state. It really makes me mad every time I think about that man. So we try not to see him anymore. James has really been through a lot for a young kid. So much of the time I worry that he's lost his childhood. I really believe that. I mean this year is the best year that he's having. He's active on weekends, he can do things, but this is the first time.

I think sometimes that I waited too long. Maybe he wouldn't have gotten so sick if I had known more about the disease before. It just never occurred to me that it could be Lyme. I feel like it's my fault sometimes. He was bitten when he was in second grade. I did everything that they told me to do, I took the tick off, I put it in a little bag, and the doctor said he was fine! I didn't know any better. They said unless he gets the rash, don't worry about it. I should have known better. Hardly anybody gets the rash. Less than 50 percent of people present with the rash. How could my doctor, the man who was protecting my child, neglect to tell me that? I'm still so angry that these doctors are so uneducated about what's happening. James never got the rash. I never saw a rash. It's been a long battle. A long one.

And I'm still fighting my own battle with all this. Sometimes, when I ask him to do things, I get this blank stare back. It's like he sees me talking, but he has no idea what I'm saying. It doesn't compute or something. And I have to stay so calm. When he says, "Mom did you just say something?" I have to say, "Yes! You were looking right at me!" It's very frustrating and hard to keep my patience. He also doesn't have too many people other than me to talk to. He doesn't have many friends. I think he feels different from other kids or something. I don't know.

I just wish that more people knew about this. If I had known, I could have prevented my baby boy from having a childhood consumed with illness. Don't other parents want to be able to do that for their children? Why wouldn't they?

CHAPTER 17

JAMES THOMAS

Seeing someone younger than I am articulate the chronic Lyme narrative was immensely powerful. At seventeen, James was obviously frustrated with his experience, but his optimism worked to mask his frustrations and hardship. He had no agenda. He was simply telling me what life was like every day, and seemed surprised by the effect his story had on his mother, his sister, and me.

The following are excerpts from his interview transcript.

It started in the middle of seventh grade, maybe a little earlier than that. I don't know, I can't remember. I had this really bad muscle achiness, and I thought maybe I had bad growing pains or something. I didn't know what it was. My muscles would do this weird shaky thing, and I just kept thinking it had to be normal. It had to be, right? Then by the end of seventh grade it became unbearable pain. I couldn't hold a pencil. I couldn't get out of bed. I was missing days of school. It was a pretty bad experience, to say the least.

My mom gave me a week that summer to just sort of lay in bed, and that's what I did. She said if I wasn't better by the end of the week we would go to a doctor. Well we saw doctor after doctor after doctor and I wasn't getting better, I was just getting worse. Finally we got my pediatrician to test me for Lyme, and I tested off-the-charts positive. So we went to see this one doctor who we just did not have a very good experience with. He put me on the normal protocol, two weeks of Doxy, and that did absolutely nothing for me. It just made me worse. So we went back to see him and he asked me, "Well, what do you think we should do about this?" I didn't know! I was twelve! He was the doctor, you know?

Anyway, then we decided to go see a new doctor and we found my current Lyme guy. He is just a great doctor, we love him. He put me on so many different oral antibiotic combinations for years, three years. I was on every single oral antibiotic he could think of, but that didn't work so I had to go on IV. I really did not want to do that. But I would just get a little better and then level off. I wasn't better yet. I wasn't all the way there. I think I got up to taking thirty-five pills a day. I hated that, and I knew I needed the IV, but I just didn't want to walk around with a nametag that said HI MY NAME IS JAMES. I'M SICK. You know? That's what it was going to be for me. I guess it was pretty cool watching the IV go in, it was like a TV show or something, but I hated it after that. It always used to get caught on things and pull on my arm. When I had that stupid machine that squeezed in medicine, the IV pump, I dropped it and it almost pulled the port out. I bled for days. It hurt so badly. The IV was just not really much fun. It got taken out about a year ago, I guess. I still wasn't better. So then we went to see this other doctor to try something new.

He did these things called Rife machines. Apparently we have these different energy tracks that run through our bodies, and are all connected. When they electrically charge one part of your body, it's supposed to come on the other side of that energy track, or channel, or whatever, if you don't have anything blocking it. Most people have about 10 percent electrical loss in a Rife machine trial, but if you have spirochetes or something blocking a specific channel, you have huge energy loss because they are just sucking up the energy. We figured out everything I had by running different electrical signals through my body. It didn't hurt or anything, it didn't shock me. The signal just goes in and out and sees where you have a problem. Then the Rife machine gets placed on top of those problem spots and sends a huge electrical signal to just blow everything up, which is pretty cool I guess, but it just wasn't for me.

I met this guy at a train station once. This old guy. He first told me about the Rife machine and said it really helped him with his Lyme disease. I don't know what this would be like, but this guy had parties at his house where people would come over and use that machine. It just wasn't for me though. It might have been with a different doctor. I don't do anything unless I really trust my doctor. That's been hard. Yeah, that's been sort of that.

I went back to see my original Lyme doctor and moved onto that butt thing. Bicillin shots. Jesus, I hated those. They just hurt a lot. I guess it was sort of fun when I got to ride around in the wheelchair at the hospital when I went to get them. Not all bad I guess. I stopped that a month ago. I didn't want to take pills anymore, you know? I couldn't. I was so tired of it. So my mom found these holistic vitamin powder things that I'm doing instead. They taste great, and I can drink them. No more pills. They're actually working too. I'm feeling better. My memory still isn't great, but I have energy to do things again. I think I'm getting really lucky with this stuff.

My mom has been such a huge help through all of this. My dad has had a pretty hard time. He just couldn't face it. So that's been difficult. It's fine but—I don't know. It's whatever. It hasn't only been hard with him. It's been hard with a lot of people. Like my pediatrician—what an idiot. He kept saying to me, "Are you sure you have Lyme?" I was just a little kid—I didn't know.

It's really nice to be able to go to school again. I haven't missed too many days of school yet this year. My hands stopped freezing up. They used to just paralyze, like rigor mortis or something. They aren't doing that anymore. I can get through the whole day of school. That's cool, because I like school a lot. The biggest issue now is the memory thing. I can deal with feeling like garbage, but my brain is just not working anymore. I went to take this processing test in the City and some parts of my brain tested in the ninety-fifth percentile and some parts tested in the first or second. The parts that are affected by the Lyme are the parts that I need for school. My grades are just garbage now. It's not because I'm not trying—I am—but my brain just can't handle it. I forget stuff. I don't remember the things I read. It's hard. I can't recall anything naturally anymore. And I used to be a really smart kid, I really did. I hate that this disease has made me sort of dumb you know?

I have a 504[45] to help me in school, but the teachers don't really help very much. They just do what they're going to do, and it's not like I'm going to go to a special-ed program or anything. If I get Cs forever then whatever, that's fine. But when I study for a test—and [then when I take] the test I don't even know what the stuff is: that really discourages me. It's hard when my teachers think I'm not trying, because I am! I'm trying so hard. I just can't remember the things they want me to do.

Most of my friends don't know really the extent that I'm sick. It's not that I've tried not to tell them. If they want to know they can, but none of my friends really seem interested in knowing the extent of it. Plus, I can't describe how I feel at all. I can say "achiness," but it's really not achiness. I call it feeling Lymey. I don't know what the words are to tell them what's happening so I haven't really tried. Now, I don't tell any new friends I have Lyme anymore. See, kids don't want to hang out with sick people. I don't want them to think I'm different right away. I already feel like that, I don't need them to make me feel even more alien.

I wish more people could understand that Lyme is a real problem. I've been trying to get *Under Our Skin* to be shown in our health classes,

I think they are going to start that next semester. I'm excited for that, but I'm also worried about it because people might not care. They might not want to care. People don't want to know what I'm feeling unless I'm feeling good. The reality of the situation is that I'm not feeling good at all, but no one wants to hear that.

It feels pretty good to say all this out loud, to feel like someone cares. I should do this more. Fingers crossed, I guess.

INTERLUDE

The documentary The Punk Singer, *about riot grrrl feminist icon Kathleen Hanna, shares in part Hanna's life-threatening experience with Lyme disease. As Dennis Bernstein writes in a* Truthout *interview with the film's director, Sini Anderson: "While filming the documentary, Sini Anderson was also diagnosed with Lyme disease, and began her own multi-year struggle for a diagnosis and treatment. She then began noticing just how many women have Lyme disease." Anderson now considers Lyme a feminist issue, and as of 2014 is interviewing women for a new documentary. She's noticed in particular the social tendency to dismiss women as exaggerating or overdramatic, and about the intense effect that dismissal has on the female experience and diagnosis of Lyme disease.[46]*

More women than men live with chronic Lyme. Anderson believes this is the result of the overwhelming tendency for women's expressions of their symptoms to be dismissed—that women must speak out again and again before they and their complaints are taken seriously. By which time, of course, Lyme disease has had ample opportunity to worsen.

I wonder if there is also a reverse effect at play here. Might the reason that more women are diagnosed with chronic Lyme be that men don't feel that they can or should articulate pain? Our rigid conception of masculinity may discourage many men from giving voice to their symptoms.

CHAPTER 18

CHRIS PATTERSON

Many of the people I interviewed struggled to speak about the most difficult moments of their illness. This was certainly the case with Chris Patterson, forty-eight, with whom I spoke by phone. I think for many people words just aren't powerful enough; it's as if the words you need to articulate your experience don't even exist.

The following are excerpts from his interview transcript.

I have to warn you, I'm a success story. I hope that's all right. So, I was first infected with Lyme in the summer of 2005. My primary symptom was a high fever, one that did not let up for two continuous weeks. I just kept thinking I'd get better, you know? I never really felt that bad. Anyway my wife eventually made me go down to the hospital, and that's where I was first diagnosed with Lyme. They said I was probably good to go and sent me to this other infectious disease doctor. If I didn't have a saint for a wife, I probably wouldn't have gone, but she made me an appointment later that day. That woman knows what she's doing. To be honest, I don't really remember my drive to the doctor. I think my fever might have been too high. I was delirious.

Anyway, that doctor basically told me that I was not fit to walk down the street and immediately checked me back into the hospital. I was there for two long nights, and three longer days. The first night they removed the tick, which had been embedded in my back for over two weeks. After three weeks of IV treatment I was better. Cured.

I really don't remember too much of it, and to be honest, it isn't the easiest thing for me to talk about. But these days, I'm feeling good. I'm putting it behind me. I could be cured. I mean that I don't think the Lyme bacteria are in my blood stream anymore. I still have some problems every once in a while. Like synonyms, I have so much trouble with synonyms. I can think of one word, but never find a word that means the same thing. The doctor says he thinks that might be from the Lyme, damage from the fever that I maintained for such a long period of time. I just think I'm getting old.

I know I'm lucky though. There are a lot of people who don't have it as easy as I did, and even still I didn't have an easy go. Here's what I really think: You want to end this epidemic? Take the antibiotics. If you feel like you have it, you do.

CHAPTER 19

MICHAEL CASHEL

I knew I needed to speak to my father about what happened to him in the years before I was fully aware of his condition. But though I'd decided to interview him, it was several months before I was strong enough to actually conduct the meeting. I had other excuses then, but I think I postponed the interview because I was unprepared to accept any part I had played in the silencing of the chronic Lyme community that was so enraging to me. It wasn't until our interview that I realized the true breadth of my own ignorance about his experience with Lyme. One of the people closest to me suffered from the same disease as I did, but for years I couldn't listen to him talk about it.

The following are excerpts from my dad's interview transcript.

I can't prove this any of this, but I think that I was infected with Lyme disease as far back as when I was sixteen years old. I spent my summers landscaping on Fishers Island, which is right across the sound from Old Lyme, and there were plenty of ticks there. I'm sure I was bit and never saw a ring, and back in the early eighties no one would have known what the ring was in any case. When I went off to college in 1980, I was in pretty good shape and played intramural soccer for my fraternity team. I would randomly wake up with my right knee massively swollen. I hadn't twisted it in a game, I hadn't fallen on it, I hadn't done anything to it, but it was so swollen that it wouldn't bend. Three days later it would be fine. Nobody could understand what that was; it was just kind of a weird oddity of me being me.

I got older. I moved in the city. In 1988 your mom and I moved to London, we started having kids, and life was grand. I used to run every day in Richmond Park when we lived in East Sheen, and they had a herd of around two thousand Roe deer when we were living there. Who knows, maybe that's where I was infected.

When we moved back to the United States I started to get sicker, but I didn't notice. I would rationalize things away. I remember going to our family doctor to talk about how I felt like I always had the flu. I couldn't get out of my own way. He tested me for Lyme disease and said I didn't have it. About three weeks went by and I was just dragging, so I went back and he tested me again. This time the results came back positive. He gave me three weeks of Doxy and said, "Take this medicine, and you're cured. Don't bother me again with this." So I didn't. I was raised in a pretty strict Irish Catholic family, and was taught not to complain. You pull your socks up, and do your work. So I pulled my socks up, and did my work.

I worked on a big trading floor for a large investment bank. There was a lot of responsibility, and that must have been tiring me out. Then I started to notice that I would walk across the trading floor to ask someone a question, and I would find myself not knowing why I was standing where I was, or who I was going to talk to. I found myself reading the same research report over and over and over again. I would read the same page, realizing three-quarters of the way through that I had already read it. I couldn't take in or retain any information. I couldn't remember anything. That was weird. I would say, "Maybe it's just that I have five little kids!" We had moved into a new house, I got up early in the morning, got home late at night, and maybe I was overtired or hungover. I started falling asleep at the wheel while driving home, so I used to drink four or five cups of coffee in the afternoon just to get myself awake enough to be able to make the drive. I would bite the insides of my cheeks until they bled to stay awake.

One night Mom took me out for dinner and she said, "You're disconnected, you are not talking to the kids, you don't talk to me, and you are always exhausted. If you can't get your shit together, I'm going to divorce you." We went home. I went into the kitchen to get a beer. I came back into the room and I said, "It was really nice to be able to spend some time with you tonight." I swear to God that I had no recollection that she had told me that she wanted to get a divorce. Absolutely none. Things were unraveling.

The next night I was driving home on the West Side Highway. I was going about sixty miles per hour and I passed out. I spun my car around twice. How I didn't hit anybody, I don't know. I woke up and realized that the wheel was locked over, and the car was spinning. I took my hands off the steering wheel, I took my foot off the brake and said, "Oh my God, I'm going to die." But then the car straightened out, and I was just driving. I had to say to myself, "Pull over, you idiot, you might have just killed someone." When I pulled over I started shaking like a leaf. I spun my car around during rush hour on the West Side Highway. I don't know how I didn't hit anyone. How I survived that I have no idea. But I did.

A couple of days later we went to a cookout at our friend's house and she had PICC line on her arm. I remember saying, "What the hell is that?" She told me it was a PICC line and that she had really bad Lyme disease. Literally every symptom she mentioned to me I had. She told me her doctor's name, it was Dr. Raxlen, and I went to see him as soon as I could. When I went, I tested positive for everything. I had all three co-infections; I had lesions on my brain, and hepatitis in my blood. He said, "It's amazing to me that you are up walking around, because you're so sick." I had no idea. You just rationalize it away.

Thank God for Dr. Raxlen. He helped us. He got us better. He had the guts to go against a lot of conventional wisdom and I will be forever grateful to him for that.

It took a while for your mom to understand everything that was happening, I think. I remember she was playing bridge with some of her friends in Greenwich and they were talking about a friend who got so sick with Lyme that she was hospitalized. I think the penny dropped for Mom then. She came rushing home and she took care of me.

I had to tell my boss at work that I was afraid my memory issues might incur a trading error for the company. They were incredibly supportive, and I took six weeks off. In my review that year though, they said they were not going to pay me and they were not going to promote me because I had been sick so much that year.

Ironically, I never had as big a year in production terms as I did that year, in spite of being sick. Soon after that conversation I realized my time was done at that firm and I left to join another one. I had been there almost ten years. Since then, I have worked at several firms trying to find my spot again; it's been a real challenge. Having said all that, you make the best of your situation. It's been a wonderful ride, but at the beginning it was pretty fucking scary. I remember one time I took the boys to a Yankee game and I was finishing my IV over one of those big garbage cans outside of Yankee stadium. I looked like a drug addict trying to shoot myself up, but I knew I had to do what I had to do to live my life.

In hindsight, the benefit for me of having Lyme and getting as sick as did was that it helped me help you get through your experience with it. I knew you needed help when I saw Lyme disease in you. Maybe I didn't help you as much as you wanted me to, but I tried. I felt that I was better able to help you because I knew what it felt like; I understood your situation because I had been through it myself. But it was so hard to watch you when you were sick. Your mom and I went through this horrible pain knowing you were in pain—it was like I could feel it for you.

Sometimes I feel like I let you down because I didn't take you to see Dr. Raxlen sooner. Do you feel like that? That's the hardest part for me; we could have taken you sooner. I don't understand how we let you get so sick when it had already happened once in our family. I feel like I let you down in that respect. I should have been more forceful; we could have taken you sooner. A lot of the reason why I didn't was because of how my own experience played out. No one thought I was sick. Mom didn't realize it until much later. Our family was a microcosm for what is happening in the nation.

I couldn't tell people at work that I was sick. When I finally did I got hurt for it, and ultimately felt that I had to leave the company. Even though the people who loved me and knew me best could see I was sick, the medical community said I was fine, so my friends and family thought so too. The same thing happened when you got sick. Your mom held on to a lot of denial because she didn't want you to experience sickness like I did. She doubted our doctors and she doubted herself. In an effort to help, her family helped turn us toward the doctors in Boston, but all they did was make one of the best parents I have ever had the privilege to know question her parenting. It was a crime.

Our own situation is endemic of the disease and the havoc it wreaks on families. The hurt and resentment of being ignored on both sides is what has so damaged our relationships. All that started and continued because of Lyme. Trust has been broken, and that is so hard to repair.

I guess we did have some great wins as a result of all this, though. We got our house in Vermont when I was really sick; some of my best, most cherished memories of my entire life come from that house. Driving up in the car and playing the tree game with you saved me. I was having medicine pumped into my body while driving to take my kids skiing, but spending that time together felt necessary for me. The love you guys gave me saved me. That's why I'll never let go of Vermont. That's where I got better. There was more love and support for me at our house in Vermont than there was anywhere else in the world. That's how I got better.

I think my relationship with Mom is getting better. We've been through countless hours of marriage counseling talking about how it's affected our family. It had a difficult impact on our relationship, but your mother is a terrific lady and we are working through it. We will for the rest of our lives. Lyme disease was a kick in the balls for us; there is no doubt about that. But there is so much love and so much respect, so I know we'll figure it out. We all will. It will get figured out.

CHAPTER 20

COMING TOGETHER

In the fall of 2012, the leaves took their time changing color. While some had already turned orange and brown, others were still as green and lush as they'd been back in August, as if they were confused, unsure of where they stood in time. The weather was similar: some days were hot like Indian summer, other days required coat just to walk to the car. On my way to class each day, I'd focus on individual trees, imagining myself moving forward and backward in time with each step.

It was my senior year of college, and I knew I should have felt empowered walking across campus, now a master of its secret paths and quirky personality. There were many moments though, when I felt entirely separate from my life there. With the same ease in which I imagined moving forward and backward in time with October's confused trees, so too I moved in and out of my college experience. Each interview I conducted— about one a week that fall—pulled me out of the student body and back into the world of chronic Lyme. And though I did feel a remarkable connection to that community, I was also sensitive to the details that separated me from it. I had been off antibiotics for over two years, and throughout that time had felt only the occasional symptom. I had been able to experience collegiate life as if I had never been touched by Lyme, yet so many of the people I spoke with still felt the effects of their disease every day. As close as I felt to them, I also felt there was a part of me wasn't wholly there. And yet whenever I returned from an interview to my healthy collegiate life, the chronic Lyme narrative still dominated my thoughts. Everything reminded me of the brave people I had met. Every time I thought of them in pain, I wished I could hold on to that pain for them, so they could feel how I was feeling, if just for a couple of minutes.

About halfway through October, one of my professors recommended I speak to a student who'd been seriously ill with Lyme before arriving at Bard that fall. She would be the first interviewee who operated in the same world as mine. There was no hiding for me at Bard. I had to be my whole self if I was going to have this meeting—and that meant embracing my Lyme life in the same place where I had worked so hard to separate from it.

When I met Zoe Winther, I realized I was sitting across the table from a girl who'd been dealt the same unfortunate deal of Lyme that I had: except without any of the support I'd had the luxury of relying on. Even today, I'm not sure I can properly articulate the strength and honesty she expressed that day.

I arranged for us to meet in one of my favorite classrooms on campus. She was thin, and had long blond hair pulled back in a tight ponytail. Her fingernails were painted dark purple, almost black, but much of the paint had chipped away, revealing light bruising beneath. Hers was a face I recognized but didn't really know. I think often about how so many of the strangers with whom we almost connect might actually understand a life of pain. We might think students who don't raise their hands to speak in class do so because they don't know the answer, but what if they don't because it hurts too much to raise that hand, like it once did for me? What cracks or stalls inside them when they try to do the things we all readily and regularly do?

As we exchanged pleasantries and filled out interview paperwork, I automatically asked her, "How are you?" She just as automatically replied, "Well, thanks." I didn't yet know that wasn't true.

"People always used to call me a hypochondriac," she started. Her light voice cut through the air with a directness I did not expect. "But in reality I think I'm just very good at understanding what is happening in my body. I have a sense for it that I was forced to learn how to trust." I looked at her face. Her makeup was thick, intentionally covering what hid underneath: color for pale cheeks and lips, concealer for the bags under her eyes. At first glance she looked healthy.

She had horrible digestion problems since she'd been about eleven or twelve. From the very first stomach pain she knew something was very wrong, but for years her pain was always dismissed as hypochondria. "Over those five years I was diagnosed with so many different things, and I hooked on to every single diagnosis, committing to it, believing it fully. It was exhausting." She had to learn quickly, and too early, that health was not a passive state: it was something she had to work toward, something to maintain. "I lost my identity to those diagnoses. Throwing myself into everything, thinking of where I could get myself. I needed to reach a moment of acceptance. I needed to accept that I did not know what was happening to me. I am where I am and I can't go back." In the late spring of her junior year of high school, eating became so agonizing it was no longer worth the effort. Her description reminded me of the pain I used to feel when my clothes rubbed against my skin, and I tried to imagine that feeling on the lining of my stomach, inside my esophagus. Her final incorrect diagnosis was anorexia. "People treated me like I was mentally ill, but I knew that there was something else wrong." It wasn't that she didn't want to eat; she was physically unable to eat. Her doctors told her that was typical in patients with advanced anorexia.

She finally received a Lyme diagnosis at the end of her junior year, and got an IV Rocephin treatment through a PICC line in her arm.

Her voice exhausted itself at this part of her story, and she picked at the polish on her nails. "I knew something was wrong. I was so nervous to start the Rocephin. I thought I might be allergic or something. I didn't know. But no one listened to me; it was like they couldn't hear me or didn't want to hear me. It turned out that I had a serious infection in my catheter and that I was allergic to the medication. It took anaphylaxis to make my parents listen to me and believe me. They didn't trust me until I was nearly dead."

I couldn't imagine not having my family's support through my experience with Lyme. My anger for whatever resistance I'd felt from them seemed excessive when I heard about Zoe's relationships. Her friendships had suffered in high school, something I also never had to face. "I learned really quickly that I shouldn't talk about Lyme in front of my friends if I wanted to keep them around. It was a taboo subject at my school. If I want people to treat me seriously, I know that I can't tell them I have Lyme. So most of my new friends here at Bard don't know about it." Zoe's closest friend from high school has stopped speaking to her. Her friend's father helped author the IDSA guidelines that prevent chronic Lyme patients from receiving treatment. When she found out about Zoe's Lyme, she cut all lines of communication—after ten years of friendship. Zoe told me this with strength. "I've learned that there are some people who are toxic people. I miss her every day, but I think she was one of them."

We sat in silence for a bit. I wanted to reach across the table and squeeze her hand, but I knew that would likely hurt her. She broke the silence saying, "That felt good." She laughed quietly to herself. "I liked that silence! I can tell you feel for me, but it doesn't feel like pity. People have really treated me profoundly awfully. Doctors turn away at the emergency room when they hear I have Lyme." She told me a story about one of these trips, in which she sat on the table in anaphylactic shock as the doctor argued with her mother over the myth of Lyme disease. "It was like he wanted me to die," she said. "I trust no one now. Especially not doctors."

She flushed underneath her makeup. "I'm convinced," she continued, "that if I was a man I would have been treated and diagnosed years ago; but I'm a woman, so I'm hysterical and finicky. It's like they can diagnose me with womanhood and that's good enough for them." She was passionate when discussing how women are treated in hospitals. When Lyme is compounded with her "diagnosis of womanhood," no one takes her seriously. No symptom she describes is taken at face value, and as a result, she can't find any doctor who she feels is completely on her side. Her passion about this is almost spiritual: a belief system she is desperate to bring to the rest of the world.

I knew that chronic Lyme is not an exclusively women's health issue, though it did appear that there were more women than men affected by the late stages of the disease. It wasn't until much later that I realized how intensely the medical establishment dismisses female health issues—which are often belittled as anxiety or other emotional problems. While I didn't feel my own experience had been dictated by gender, I knew it played a large role in the medical outcomes of people like Zoe Winthers and Charlotte Lerman.

In a famous study published in the *Journal of Law, Medicine and Ethics,* "The Girl Who Cried Pain: A Bias Against Women in the Treatment of Pain," Diane E. Hoffmann and Anita J. Tarzian set out to explore the paradox of why, even though "in general, women report more severe levels of pain, more frequent incidences of pain, and pain of longer duration than [do] men," women are "nonetheless treated for pain less aggressively." In particular, they wanted to know if men and women experience pain differently and what accounts for the differences in the pain treatment they receive.[47] As Laurie Edwards states in her *New York Times* article "The Gender Gap in Pain," the researchers found that "women were less likely to receive aggressive treatment when diagnosed, and were more likely to have their pain characterized as 'emotional,' 'psychogenic,' and therefore 'not real.'"[48]

This phenomenon can have a disastrous effect on female patients of Lyme. For example, a friend of my first interviewee, Melissa Edwards, was diagnosed with a psychological imbalance, checked into a mental hospital, and treated with mood-altering medications for over two years before she was properly diagnosed and treated for Lyme. But women with "mysterious" or difficult-to-diagnose conditions aren't the only ones affected by this bias. Another study, conducted by scientists at the University of North Carolina, screened over 1.1 million patients from 1994 to 2006 and showed that, though fewer women than men have heart attacks, women are more likely to die of cardiac arrest because they are significantly less likely to get the immediate treatment they needed. "Doctors may not take women's health issues seriously," says Dr. Suzanne Steinbaum, director of Women's Heart Health at Lenox Hill Hospital in New York and an American Heart Association spokeswoman. "Women are coming in saying they're nauseous, they're fatigued, they're sweating, and doctors say, 'You're fine. It's anxiety, and it's all in your head.'"[49]

That last phrase infects the experience of so many of the patients I've spoken to about chronic Lyme. "It's all your head" is a sentiment that has changed the course of many lives, derailing the further exploration that could have saved them and their families years of pain and struggle. If we accept as truth that women are more likely than men to be dismissed as anxious or finicky, what happens when that prejudice is combined with the prejudice and doubt associated with Lyme disease? Are the two sentiments permanently entangled?

Since her diagnosis, Zoe has received forty-five different treatments. A series of doctors have given up on her, and she has lost hope that effective treatment for her even exists. The spirochetes regularly compromise her system enough to trigger within her new, life-threatening allergies—and perhaps the only treatment left to her requires months in the ICU. "So I had to take a year at college before that, you know?" she said, trying to smile. "I wanted to see what all the fuss was about. I've loved it so far. It's been wonderful. I'm happy to have this time, because I don't know what's in store for me. Every doctor thinks that college will probably kill me. People die from this disease and its complications, I think I'll probably be . . ." Her voice trailed off. "I just don't see a light at the end of this tunnel."

Zoe then got a call from her father, who was bringing the inhaler she'd left at home. She was relieved that she hadn't needed it yet, since her parents hadn't been able to deliver it until then. She rushed out to meet her dad, leaving me alone to tidy up, erasing any evidence of our meeting. Most people at Bard didn't know Zoe was as sick as she was. No one knew that she might not make it through to graduation without a stay in the ICU. My hands shook as I picked up our non-disclosure agreement, overwhelmed by the weight it seemed to carry.

When I walked outside again I saw Zoe arguing with her father through his car window. When she turned around and saw me I waved, but she did not wave back. It seemed we had gone back to being strangers, that her need to not be associated with her medical history was as strong as my own.

Back in my own car I started to cry, almost silently, muffled by anger and grief. I called my mom, who picked up halfway through the first ring as though she'd known I'd call. I didn't say much, only that I met a girl who might die from Lyme because people hadn't believed her. She listened to me cry for Zoe, for the other women I'd interviewed, for her, for myself. She listened to me just breathing, my head resting against the steering wheel, the doors locked—all while college life, blissfully unaware, buzzed around me.

Violence has never been a familiar impulse to me. But during that call with my mom I slammed my hands against the car windows and steering wheel. I thrashed against the seatbelt as if it were intentionally strapping me down. Mom kept saying this was healthy; it was all part of the grieving process. My sadness was turning to anger, into a fierce desire to do something more than just listen.

I drove home, still crying. I felt paralyzed by my anger, overwhelmed by the breadth of hardship and pain I'd vicariously lived through that fall. I felt I was getting lost in the voices and stories I'd been told; they had so filled my consciousness I could no longer hear my own thoughts. I'd heard all I felt I could bear.

All the same, I completed the few interviews that had already been scheduled. After the last one, conducted before Thanksgiving, I hoped to feel a sense of relief in the completion, a chance to catch my breath again. Instead I felt the opposite.

While I'd never told anyone I interviewed that I thought I was cured, for while I truly felt I had beaten this disease. With everyone I interviewed who still struggled with their illness, I felt guilty that I was healthy when they were still sick

It was hard for me to acknowledge when my short-term memory started to cloud, or when my language once again began to stall. I pushed aside these apparent non-symptoms as grief for those I was speaking with. I tried to ignore the pain building again in my body.

So, yes, the spirochetes started regaining control in me that December; by January 2013 I realized they were too strong for me to fight without treatment. But this time when I entered battle I didn't feel I was fighting alone. This time I had a new understanding of the support I received from my family. And I had the support of many Lyme patients who could understand and empathize with my experience as I had understood and empathized with theirs.

It's been over a year now since I first met Zoe, Melissa, Laura, James, his mother, and the others I spoke with that fall. Since then I've experienced the full cycle of illness and health; many of them have as well. Every day that I wake up and feel pain, or think of others in pain, I return to this story—hoping to draw closer to those residing in both my worlds: the world of the sick and the world of the healthy.

PART III

STRUCTURES OF SILENCE

After dedicating more than a year to chronic Lyme, I still felt overwhelmed by its complexity, by all I didn't and perhaps wouldn't ever understand. Throughout I knew I'd eventually need to speak with the experts of the Lyme world—to ask their thoughts on the science and politics of the chronic Lyme debate. But when the time came to immerse myself in their world and to learn their language, I wasn't sure where to start.

To follow are the voices of people who know Lyme disease almost as well as those who live with it; their perspectives influence and shape the living experience of chronic Lyme patients every day.

CHAPTER 21

DETOUR

I'm the type of person who likes everything to get worked out in the end, every narrative tidily wrapped up and neatly tied in a bow. This applies as much to stories of others as to my own. So after I conducted my last Lyme interview at the end of April 2013, I used some interviews and small sections of memoir to build my senior thesis at Bard. Upon graduation, I fully anticipated walking away from that apparently complete articulation of my experience. Though I'd been sick again that winter and spring, I'd simply pushed through it, as I'd done in the past, expecting life to then return to normal—expecting that this time was the last time, that now for certain I had defeated the disease.

Immediately after graduation I landed a job working for a very progressive advertising agency and got an apartment in Manhattan—ready to fully embrace life as the twenty something New Yorker I'd convinced myself I was supposed to be. I was healthy. I left no room for sickness in my New York identity.

Of course, I soon realized that everything wasn't tied in a perfect little package, that I didn't actually have a clear understanding of chronic Lyme, nor of myself in relation to Lyme. My journey toward patient advocacy felt far from over. There was still more to learn about the experience of these patients—and, though I struggled to admit it, there was clearly still more to reconcile about my own experience as well. To no one's surprise but my own, I quit my job after just one month to continue my work and research with Lyme; and again, to no one's surprise but my own, that decision was met with enthusiasm and encouragement.

There was a major facet of the living experience of chronic Lyme disease that I had yet to tackle. When immersed in the stories I collected, I fully believed they were adequate proof of chronic infection. But outside of that world, I feared they'd do nothing to change opinion—especially since much of the mainstream medical community often seems blind and deaf to patient suffering. Despite the countless stories and voices rallying behind me, I still felt silenced.

I knew we needed to change the way people talk about Lyme. But to transform the way we discuss illness in the physical world, I would have immerse myself in the more abstract ideological world. That space terrified me. I knew how to sit with fellow patients to discuss their emotional and physical understandings of their illnesses; and we always entered the conversation with a mutual understanding of its purpose. But outside the world of patient narratives, the conversation isn't so simple. In order for me to understand and ultimately challenge the resistance to accepting the chronic Lyme narrative as an infectious disease—not a psychological one—I'd need to speak to those who informed that resistance, those whose politics and perspective make Lyme a disease unlike any other.

I refer, of course, to the scientists and doctors who firmly trust the CDC's treatment guidelines. But entering into conversation with them scared me on several levels. They not only knew more than I did, but they also heartily disagreed with me. I had already been crippled by losing my sense of certainty about my physical illness—I didn't want to experience that again. How could I possibly view their perspectives objectively, given that experience? It was naïve, but to me, the story of chronic Lyme had always been one of good versus evil, of ignorance versus enlightenment, of the weak versus the strong. If I knew where I fit in a community of people oppressed by the medical system; how could I even consider speaking to one of its oppressors?

Before I decided to write about Lyme, I met with Professor Robert Kelly at Bard and shared these concerns. Professor Kelly looked at me, leaned forward in his chair, and placed his large, aged, ringed fingers on my knees. "Just talk to them, Allie," he said. "You're making walls where walls don't exist. We're all human. Just talk to them."

I had tried to leave my story of chronic illness behind me when I entered the world beyond college. But, in truth, my journey into the narrative of Lyme had only just begun.

CHAPTER 22

IN THE LINE OF FIRE: DR. EUGENE SHAPIRO

Quick internet searches of "The Clinical Assessment, Treatment, and Prevention of Lyme Disease, Human Granulocytic Anaplasmosis, and Babesiosis: Clinical Practice Guidelines," reveal the potent hatred that much of the chronic Lyme community holds for the authors of the IDSA treatment guidelines for Lyme. These authors are depicted as traitors: to their own profession, to the patients they are meant to treat. Their guidelines prevent many patients from receiving the treatment they need, thus extensively prolonging their suffering—and thus proving that how we speak about illness vastly influences the way those afflicted will experience it.

I reached out to each member of the IDSA committee, some of them repeatedly. One of the first I tried was Dr. Gary Wormser. As he is based out of Mount Kisco, New York, just a few miles from my childhood home, his name surfaced many times throughout my childhood treatments and diagnoses of Lyme disease. To me, he was the epitome of doctors who dismiss the existence of a chronic Lyme infection, and I had long before dismissed out of hand his stance in the matter. Of course, in so doing I was guilty of the same act I hated him for, but for a long time my anger prevented me from seeing that. As it turned out, I wouldn't need to try to respect his half of our conversation; he never granted me one.

Of the fourteen guidelines contributors I contacted, only one responded: Dr. Eugene Shapiro. A professor of General Pediatrics and of Epidemiology at Yale, Dr. Shapiro is also a resident physician and pediatric infectious disease specialist at Yale–New Haven Hospital; in addition he is the Associate Chair for Clinical Translational Educational Research at Yale and Chair of the American Board of Pediatrics. He is best known in the chronic Lyme community for actively promoting the IDSA guidelines in his own practice and opinions.

Before Dr. Shapiro and I met in person, we exchanged a series of emails in which he shared some of the notes he'd received from the "so-called chronic Lyme community," as he put it. The messages were toxic— the anger and hate contained in each was overwhelming. One read: "How can you sleep at night?" Another proposed that Nazi physician Dr. Joseph Mengele, who conducted horrific experiments on Jews at Auschwitz, would have admired his work.

We also spoke by phone before we met. I started to explain my research to Dr. Shapiro, and stated that I was exploring the Lyme controversy—

"Controversy?" he interrupted.

"Well yes, a lot of people believe that Lyme can persist in the body even after years of antibiotic treatment."

"True," he retorted. "A lot of people also believe that God created the world in seven days."

Given that response, I worried he would be so rigid, so disenchanted, that an open and honest conversation would be impossible. I entered our meeting with a sense of apprehension. In fact, it was surprising to me that I even followed through with our appointment. But as soon as we met his famed villain persona started to fade.

I was waiting for him outside a coffee shop in New Haven, and when he arrived he quickly ushered me in out of the cold. He bought me a cup of tea, offering breakfast as well, and thanked me for coming before I had a chance to thank him for the same. He told me about his granddaughter and his children long before we started speaking about Lyme.

Dr. Shapiro studied English and psychiatry in school; he didn't originally plan on becoming a physician. But in the 1990s he developed an interest in infectious disease pediatrics, subsequently studied at the University of California, San Francisco. When he started practicing pediatrics, one of his children was bitten by a tick. That bite made Shapiro aware of the gross lack of information surrounding Lyme disease, and fueled his desire to "find the answer" to that mystery.

Less than ten years later, in 2000, he'd developed enough of a professional reputation to be asked to contribute to the IDSA treatment guidelines—the participation of which has since earned him a more infamous reputation in the Lyme community.

Dr. Shapiro told me about the effect this dual reputation has on treating new patients: essentially, it's gotten to the point that he first has to perform an "internet-dectomy" to discount not only the slander against him but also some of the "bogus" information that "too many patients of Lyme disease" happen upon during their internet research.

Shapiro took the time to specify why the claims against him and the IDSA committee are false. "Look," he said, "if this disease was impossible to cure, that would be good for me. I'd get more money, that'd be good. The idea that we were somehow paid off for those guidelines . . . makes no sense. They are simply guidelines, we didn't have a vested interest in the results." He went on to clarify that he'd also never been "paid off" for the numerous times he'd testified as an expert witness. Though I hadn't asked him anything about bribes or financial involvement, it was clear that people regularly brought up these issues. "It's the other doctors who are making the money," he continued. "Most of them don't take insurance. They take hundreds of dollars out of patients' pockets for every visit."

"When you say 'other doctors,'" I asked, "you are referring to doctors who treat patients past the IDSA's recommended course of treatment?"

"Right. Some people call them 'Lyme-literate.' They are the guys who are on board with a chronic Lyme diagnosis."

"I've read a bit about your thoughts on what's going on with patients who continue to feel the symptoms of Lyme after their diagnosis—but can you speak to that?"

Dr. Shapiro encouraged me to go back and look at other historical medical phenomena, like chronic mono (mononucleosis), which he said many people suffered from until chronic Lyme came along. "There have always been different labels for the same issue," he stated, "and those labels have simply changed with the times." Dr. Shapiro believes that patients dealing with the symptoms of chronic Lyme disease are not dealing with an infection in their body, but instead are dealing with something called, "medically unexplained symptoms," also referred to as a "functional somatic syndrome." And chronic Lyme is not the only syndrome that falls into this category—chronic fatigue syndrome and irritable bowel syndrome also are categorized by patients dealing with medically unexplained symptoms. There is no serological explanation these patients suffering, yet they still suffer.

It was a strange moment: sharing a conversation with a doctor who, like many others, is convinced that my medical experience did not have a physiological basis. He didn't point a finger at me; he didn't even refer to any of those suffering from chronic Lyme disease as dealing with something that's all in their heads. Instead, he offered an explanation that was disturbingly difficult to poke a hole in.

He is of the belief that chronic Lyme, and other manifestations of "medically unexplained symptoms," are part of a social phenomenon, a pattern that has repeated over hundreds of years. While there is no physical explanation for the symptoms people experience, no one denies that the symptoms are real. Patients do feel what they say they feel: it's just that those symptoms aren't caused by an active infection. It's a "medically un-explained" phenomenon, which is best treated with pain management and therapy. While Dr. Shapiro's theory does not suppose that these patients feel healthy, it does attribute the feelings of illness to the patients themselves rather than to an infection. In other words, just because patients can convincingly describe their suffering doesn't mean they're actually dealing with infectious disease.

Who was I to say that this theory was wrong? Any feelings of certainty I had could easily be debunked as part of this supposed phenomenon. As someone who experiences these "medically unexplained symptoms" myself, of course I empathize with others who've shared my experience. And, not only does that empathy validate and justify my feelings of illness, it also justifies the empathy of others. What if we were just fueling each other's fire?

From that standpoint, the classification of Lyme patients as "malin-gerers" makes sense, as the diagnosis seems to have more to do with the patient's personality or psyche than it does with what's actually going on in the patient's body. But why is it, then, that so many people have such similar experiences? It was hard to believe that a single social phenom-enon brought people across varying countries and cultures to experience the same symptoms. And what of the patients living in countries where doctors have never even heard of Lyme: how did they manage to psycho-logically concoct symptoms they'd never seen presented in anyone else?

As I looked to the literature in an attempt to better understand it, I found that patients were often grouped together in social groups, but that these groupings did not account for many of the people suffering from per-sistent Lyme. In their article "Assessment and Management of Medically Unexplained Symptoms," Dr. Simon Hatcher and Dr. Bruce Arroll ask, "Who gets medically unexplained symptoms?" Their answer:

"The most consistent finding is that people with medically unexplained symptoms have fewer years of formal education than the general population. A case control study found that experiencing a parental illness or lack of care in childhood predisposes women to the development of medically unexplained symptoms as adults."

The article also states:

"Clinical presentations vary greatly—from people who frequently attend the general practitioner with minor symptoms to people with chronic fatigue who are bedbound. What unites them, however, is the difficulty in explaining the presenting symptoms on the basis of any known pathology. Strong feelings are common, with patients often referred to in pejorative terms as 'frequent fliers,' 'heart sink patients,' 'thick folder patients,' or 'somatisers.' Doctors may feel that their competence is challenged by their inability to explain the symptoms, and patients may feel that they are disbelieved and accused of fabricating their symptoms."[50]

While I was familiar with the patient frustration described here, the patient body within the article did not match the patients I knew.

Another article, by Dr. Leonard H. Sigal et al., offers additional patient descriptions:

"As many as half the patients presenting to Lyme disease specialty clinics are depressed and/or suffering from excessive stress. Excessive stress and depression may be due to having a chronic illness; alternatively, it is possible that depression and high levels of stress may have preceded the initial infection and are symptomatic of an underlying vulnerability, which predisposes to chronic, nonspecific symptoms and complaints."

The article also states:

"Acceptance of the diagnosis of chronic Lyme disease provides a number of benefits for these sufferers. It legitimizes the pain, suffering, and disability. It provides a structure by which to understand a very frightening experience. It produces a community with which to identify and from which to draw strength and comfort. It gives the sufferer a means by which to address the suffering on personal and societal levels."[51]

Dr. Arthur J. Barsky and Dr. Jonathan F. Borus similarly describe this patient body:

"Patients with functional somatic syndromes have explicit and highly elaborated self-diagnoses, and their symptoms are often refractory to reassurance, explanation, and standard treatment of symptoms. They share similar a phenomenology, high rates of co-occurrence, similar epidemiologic characteristics, and a higher-than-expected prevalence of psychiatric comorbidity. Although discrete pathophysiologic causes may ultimately be found in some patients with functional somatic syndromes, the suffering of these patients is exacerbated by a self-perpetuating, self-validating cycle in which common, endemic, somatic symptoms are incorrectly attributed to serious abnormality, reinforcing the patient's belief that he or she has a serious disease."[52]

It seems that the unifying description of this diagnosis does not convey what is actually happening in the body, but rather how patients deal with what they are experiencing. So while this diagnosis classifies patients such that they are treated psychologically, it does not enable doctors to treat patients' physical symptoms.

This, of course, was familiar to me, and as I recalled my reaction to my own psychological diagnosis, I asked him, "When you describe this diagnosis to your patients, what is their reaction normally like?"

"Well, most of the patients we see are not the patients that are angry conspiracy theorists. Otherwise they wouldn't show up to see us in the first place. You know? They go to Dr. Jones." Dr. Jones was a name that had surfaced in a few of my interviews; like Dr. Horowitz or Dr. Raxlen, he was considered a hero by many of his patients. Dr. Shapiro continued: "But how do I speak to them about all this? You know, it really depends. I'm going to see a patient on Friday who is pretty committed to chronic Lyme disease, and that will affect the way we talk about this. It depends on who they are. You try to find out what their questions are, and what their understanding is before you enter the conversation. I try to figure out if they are intelligent enough to understand—well, no—I try to figure out what their beliefs are and what they are thinking, and then I try to explain what Lyme disease is and what it isn't. You know, I tell them the truth. One of the big things is that you have to validate them. What you don't want to say is that it's all in your head, it's all bullshit."

"Because then they are immediately going to feel dismissed."

"Exactly, which they do sometimes anyway. It's funny—if you go online, you can Google doctors and you can see their ratings and health grades. People who have never seen me write all these horrible things about me. I have horrible grades. I mean, I know it's all bullshit. These people have never seen me."

"Does that ever influence your own patients' understandings of you?"

"No. I've realized that you really need to validate what's going on. If a patient is really locked in to Lyme disease, I say, 'Look you've already been treated adequately for Lyme six times over. There has never been a strain of the bacteria that is resistant to an antibiotic. There is no such thing as resistance.' I have some people who have been on antibiotics for a year, and the day they stop it they believe their symptoms come back. I try to explain how that doesn't make sense in terms of physiology, but it's more important sometimes to validate the symptoms. We don't really know exactly what's causing it. And so many of the patients will get bogus lab results, so we can't really prove they have it. Patients will come in with one band on the Western blot and say that they are positive."

I next adopted a different angle. "Your interest in pediatrics is very interesting to me. What do you think about kids who continue to display symptoms for long periods of time—do you think their parents play a role in that? And if you do, what's that role?"

"There is a wide spectrum on this issue but it's pretty clear. If you're a kid and you say, 'I have a pain in my knee,' and your parent says, 'Okay, here take a Tylenol and go play,' or they say, 'Oh my God! Where? How does it hurt? We need to go to the doctor!'—the kid will feel differently. The parent reaction is very important. A lot of parents have anxiety, and it affects their children. I can't tell you how many parents of really severe cases are divorced and fighting, you know, custody battles, sad stuff. If you think about it, what is a better vehicle for parental anxiety than this? You have this bug that is so small you can't see it, and it's going to suck your child's blood. In the process it's going to transmit an infection that could have any manifestation known to man, and unless you're hypervigilant to detect it, it's going to ruin your child's life forever. That's how people think of this. So, it's not unusual for parents to build it up in their child's brain. It's not just Lyme disease. There are plenty of kids from parents with marital problems who come in with other symptoms. Lyme is just a convenient diagnosis that people have now."

I was somewhat surprised by the fairly standard nature of Shapiro's responses. Nothing he said seemed particularly revolutionary, or even out of the ordinary. I expected him to stand out, but his thoughts seemed reflective of everything his peers had been saying for the past ten years. I moved on to my last question.

"As you've developed your understanding of this disease," I started, "you've heard so many people tell you that you are wrong. "Have you personally, as an individual, ever doubted your own thoughts about it? Or have you always stayed confident?"

"Well, you know, when I first started out I needed to know more. So I was less confident on day one than I am now. My son actually said once, 'Dad, what if you're wrong about Lyme?'" The doctor laughed, punctuating his sentence.

"Yeah, of course," I pushed. "But, has that ever changed your thoughts and understanding of your own work?"

"No," he replied, shaking his head. "I haven't really." He made eye contact with me across the table and then looked back down into his coffee like he hoped to find something there. He was taking his time on this. "I mean, I might have changed a little bit. I've come to appreciate more the reality of the symptoms, and the destructive effect doctors can have on transmitting to patients their own feelings of frustration or inadequacy for not being able to help. Twenty years from now we might figure out all these patients have some gene, which makes them more susceptible to such and such. I mean there is a biochemical explanation for all behavior, right? There may be factors that are predisposed that we haven't identified. But what I'm very confident about, and this hasn't changed, is this is not an ongoing active infection. I'm certain about that."

I had come face-to-face with one of the villains of my story, but he hadn't lived up to my expectation. He may have been stubborn and old-fashioned, but he clearly didn't want to hurt anyone. His greatest shortcoming was his inability to admit that he could possibly be wrong.

CHAPTER 23

MIDDLE GROUND: DOCTORS OSTFELD AND KEESING

Though in meeting Dr. Shapiro I hadn't met Lyme's Dr. Mengele, I had discovered something that scared me. While Dr. Shapiro was not an evil man, his opinions were so disturbingly rigid that I worried it would be impossible for leaders of the chronic Lyme debate to ever speak to each other without prejudice. When discussing Dr. Jones, a celebrated doctor in the Lyme community, Shapiro spoke with disdain. He saw the people who went to see Dr. Jones as "conspiracy theorists," not patients simply seeking to lessen their pain. In turn, the patients who revile Dr. Shapiro use similar, if not stronger, hyperbolic language when describing him.

As to my own view: I consider Dr. Shapiro's approach to chronic Lyme disease dismissive and damaging; I won't pretend otherwise. But it in speaking to him I truly felt he had no intention to hurt. It's simply that his perspective has been pushed so far away from the perspectives of the "Lyme-literate" that it seems there is no middle ground. Is it possible for these opposite and opposing parties to understand each other, or is the landscape too polarized for any sort of mutual recognition? While I hoped I might help bridge the large gap of the chronic Lyme debate, I feared my own bias so securely planted me on one side that I'd be unable to journey toward the other without carrying a white flag.

There are those, however, who work with Lyme outside the line of fire. I like to think they operate in a more objective space, free from the burden of debate. They can offer insight on how we can bring to the foreground the patient experience of this disease, and how we can bring closer together the polarized ends of the chronic Lyme spectrum.

While living in Dutchess County, which consistently reports some of the highest rates of Lyme infection worldwide, I was surrounded by scientists and thinkers who worked closely with Lyme, and who potentially occupied this type of space. It was only after I'd moved that I found the courage to speak to them about their work.

Disease ecologist Dr. Richard Ostfeld received his PhD from UC Berkeley in 1985. He has worked closely with Lyme since joining the Cary Institute of Ecosystem Studies in Millbrook, New York, in the early 1990s, where he focuses on risk and prevention of vector-borne diseases. In 1997 Dr. Felicia Keesing also received her PhD from UC Berkeley. She is a professor of biology at Bard College and conducts her own research at the Cary Institute. Together, she and Dr. Ostfeld developed a conceptual model they call the dilution effect, which suggests that when the potential number of tick hosts increases, the risk of Lyme disease goes down. In other words, investing in biodiversity in our forests would actually protect human health.

The scientists live with their two children just outside of Bard College. Though I babysat for them during my senior year, during that time we hardly spoke about Lyme. I interviewed them via Skype in November 2013.

Dr. Ostfeld first explained that, since their work operates somewhat outside the chronic Lyme debate, they have a unique perspective on the conversation as a whole. "What Felicia and I work on is upstream from that controversy," he said. "It's about what gives a patient Lyme disease, whereas most of the controversy, although not all of it, is focused downstream. The focus is on how many patients are really sick, how long are they sick, and whether or not they are sick after they get treatment. One positive thing about having our work focused upstream is that this focus is on risk. We ask, Where do the ticks come from? Where do they get infected? What is your likelihood of coming in contact with one? Questions like this help our research feed into prevention. Everyone, people on all sides of this debate, agree that prevention is really important. Everybody loves it. In some way, we have almost immediate respect from the orthodox specialists and the patient advocates. They revile each other, but seem to respect us."

"We can talk to both groups," he continued. "We aren't immediately being written off. Because we work so firmly in the realm of statistics and evidence, we stay close to the science and avoid basing our studies on weaker levels of epistemology like anecdotes. Orthodox scientists respect our approach and see us as akin to them. On the other hand, we're in a unique position to evaluate their science, which has some serious weaknesses, and we're aware of the ways in which bias can enter into science. Scientists are human just like anyone else. Our perspectives influence the way we interpret science and data. So, we can see bias and problems with the orthodox medical professionals in such a way that the people who revile the orthodox see us as having more substance and rigor than the orthodox, whose science is often lacking in rigor, to be quite honest. I think we both see our position as one that we can help find areas of agreement and common ground. There are areas we will never find agreement, but perhaps we can reframe the questions so that we can help those patients who feel abandoned feel as though their concerns are being met."

"Do you feel that bias affects your work with Lyme?"

"Well, I would say that we personally don't have a dog in the fight about chronic Lyme," he said plainly. "So I would say the major controversies about the diagnosis and treatment of Lyme have no impact on the way we do our research. Honestly though, if you are engaged in the public world of Lyme in any way the controversy is inescapable. And, of course, we are engaged in our own controversies on the ecological side, because some of the things we've found are things that not everyone agrees with."

Objectivity in the Lyme world, Ostfeld was quick to remind me, is very hard to come by.

At this point Dr. Keesing joined in. "There is also a big gap between our science and the patient experience. As scientists, we can talk statistics, but that doesn't really help people who are trying to figure out how to make themselves better. We can talk prevention, but that doesn't help people who are already living with the disease. They are a data point. I don't mean to say that trivially, but in our work they are. And it's difficult for us to try and bridge that gap by converting our data into something relevant to their experience."

"You might think that would be unnecessary," added Dr. Ostfeld, "but it's impossible to keep yourself separate from the patient experience in our line of work. It's everywhere. And not being an expert on diagnosis and treatment doesn't rule anyone out from having an opinion."

Bias influences even the most basic actions. Reading a graph or looking at numbers may appear like an act unaffected by opinion, but too often we see what we want to see. If something suits our goal, that's what we select from the data. It was clear that Dr. Ostfeld felt that bias was a part of much of the science around him, but he also seemed to feel somewhat above that bias. Though his work may not deal with the heart of the debate, it didn't mean that debate didn't affect him. He said himself—it's inescapable.

The collective understanding of science and medicine has an enormous effect on how we live our lives. Scientists, doctors, official guidelines contributors: their decisions hugely impact entire populations. Which in essence means that we're all subject to the biases of those considered authorities in their fields. And, the more polarized the field, the more potent will be the impact of those who operate from either end.

"There is so often an epistemological disconnect in what people believe and what is actually going on. It's not exclusive to Lyme; this pervades the way people understand probability and their own personal experience. Humans are incredibly bad at understanding risk."

"We are," Dr. Keesing agreed. "And it's so much worse when we are scared. It's one thing to evaluate risk when we're going to be late to work—we aren't very good at that either—but when we're terrified we latch on to things. When we most need to be able to assess risk, that's when we are most incapable of doing it."

"Can we talk a little bit about that fear?" I asked. "A lot of people seem to avoid talking about chronic Lyme, coming down on one side or the other, because they say the science to prove it is not there. Would you say that is the case? Or do most people just not know about the science that already exists?"

"There is a huge amount known about Lyme disease," Ostfeld replied, contradicting the belief of many in the patient community. "This is one of those situations where people are fighting to be right. That is clearly the case on both sides of the chronic Lyme controversy. As a result, the major players in the debate use tactics that intentionally confuse the end users of the information. They try to undermine the opposition and bolster their own arguments in order to win, not in order to get closer and closer to the truth. There is a huge amount of information, but we lack honest brokers that are putting it out there in a transparent way. It's not that the information isn't out there, it's just that it's controversial." "Lyme disease is a great educating moment," Dr. Keesing said. "When people want to understand Lyme, they need to understand how science works. They need answers to questions like, What should I do? But trying to get answers out of the Lyme system can be very frustrating, whereas trying to get answers about how the way an antibiotic responds to another pathogen is not frustrating at all. I think there are various reasons for that. One of them connects to a larger issue in science—there are really only a couple of ways that scientists can answer questions. One of them is to do experiments, which everyone knows about. Another one is where we have correlations, like patients who take this medicine tend do better or patients who eat cabbages tend to do better than patients who don't. But we didn't experimentally give them these cabbages—we just found this correlation. It's just a pattern that you can observe. The third thing we have is to use models, which are simplifications of the system that make it easier for us to answer the question, but they are deliberately simplifications. You'll never know if you get an answer from a model, but you don't know if the conclusion you draw from that simpler version of reality will scale up to the more complicated version. Is a mouse good enough to represent humans in this way? They may well not be. So the problem is, we can't do what we want.

"We all want to do experiments with Lyme, because then we can isolate cause and effect, but in order to do the experiments that we want, we'd have to take a bunch of people who don't have Lyme and give half of them Lyme, and then half of those we'd treat with something and then the other half we wouldn't. Then we'd see if the people who weren't treated developed chronic Lyme. Obviously we can't do that because that's completely unethical. So we're giving infections to mice, because we can infect mice or some other model. The problem is that we're doing those experiments in models and they can't scale up. We're trapped; what we all want to do, if we really want to answer the question in the way that no one can argue with, is the kind of experiment that no one can do, so we're left with all these imperfect versions."

"And because this is a societal issue where people are invested in a specific answer," Ostfeld added, "they can use the imperfections of the model to their benefit, and further their claims rather than seek the truth."

In other words: objectivity in the chronic Lyme debate may be unobtainable.

CHAPTER 24

THE PATH FORWARD: DR. RICHARD HOROWITZ

In August 2012, at the very start of my senior year at Bard, I visited the Kagyu Thubten Chling Monastery to meet with John Fallon, a nurse practitioner who works alongside Dr. Richard Horowitz, one of the most famous Lyme physicians in America. This marked my first foray into researching chronic Lyme. Walking under the Tibetan prayer flags flanking the entrance, I felt as though I'd entered someone's secret, nestled in a forest. Though I'd normally feel nervous for a meeting this this, somehow my anxiety evaporated in this space, which seemed to have its own pulse, its own breath.

After sharing a meal with Mr. Fallon and a group of resident monks, John and I walked the grounds. Looking up at the many massive sculptures throughout the monastery, I remember feeling strangely like I shared a sense of pilgrimage with those worshiping around me. And as I shared more with John about my own work and research, the words tumbling out of my mouth felt electric. I was excited about Lyme in a way I had never felt before.

As we made our way through the grounds, John—occasionally stopping to move worms that had crawled onto the pavement after the recent rain—spoke calmly about his patients, many of whom had been sick with tick-borne infections for much of their lives. He answered my questions and shared stories of his colleague, Dr. Richard Horowitz, including some of the political struggles the world-renown physician had faced earlier in his practice. Based on his work with thousands of patients, Dr. Horowitz was then in the process of writing a book, which John imagined would definitively state how the medical world should be dealing with and thinking about complex tick-borne illnesses.

Over a year later, in the late fall of 2013, I used that book, *Why Can't I Get Better? Solving the Mystery of Lyme and Chronic Disease,* released just weeks before, to prepare for my interview with Dr. Horowitz.

Dr. Richard Horowitz is the medical director of the Hudson Valley Healing Arts Center based out of Hyde Park, New York. The integrative medical center combines traditional and more contemporary approaches for the treatment of Lyme and other tick-borne illnesses. In the past few decades Dr. Horowitz has seen over twelve thousand patients, who travel from around the world seeking his guidance. Though many have been sick for years, a large percentage complete his treatment feeling healthy. Dr. Horowitz is also one of the founding members of ILADS, the International Lyme and Associated Diseases Society, as well as past president of the ILADEF, the International Lyme and Associated Diseases Educational Foundation.

"I'm sorry I'm a bit late." Dr. Richard Horowitz shook my hand hurriedly and offered me a chair. He had come straight from an interview with NPR, explaining the "radio announcer just would not stop chattering." It was strange to be sitting in his office. I had read so much about him that I'd never thought of him as an individual—only as an idea.

"So is this a school paper or something?" he asked.

"It started as that," I replied, "but I'm actually developing my own manuscript that I hope will be published soon."

"Oh! Good for you."

I struggled to read his tone—beyond that he was pressed for time. I assured him I had just a few questions.

"Patient narratives are the real backbone of the project I'm working on now—talking through people's experiences. Many of them struggle to understand why this disease is so readily dismissed as psychological or emotional. I'd like to focus on that. Do you consider this widespread dismissive attitude an issue specific to chronic Lyme disease?"

"I think it's both. I think chronic illness is misunderstood, but the problem specifically with Lyme is that the blood testing is not very reliable. Doctors are heavily relying on blood tests to make the diagnosis. If you go into a doctor's office, and you tell them you're tired, you're not sleeping, you're anxious or depressed, the doctor will likely call it chronic fatigue or fibromyalgia—that's assuming they've even thought to do a Lyme test. Oftentimes they'll do the ELISA test, which will come back negative, and they don't know to do the Western blot. What so many doctors don't realize is that there are one hundred strains of Lyme in the United States, and three hundred strains worldwide. This is not a disease you're going to be able to pick up from just one blood test. The issue is that we are thinking of it too simplistically. It's much more complex than many physicians may think."

This idea of complexity and multiplicity drives Dr. Horowitz's practice. One of the biggest problems he sees in standard treatment practices for the disease is considering Lyme a single infection without any other contributing factors. Without treating those other factors, infections, and imbalances, patients will not get better.

Not surprisingly, this multiplicity model plays a dominant role in his book as well. *Why Can't I Get Better? Solving the Mystery of Lyme and Chronic Disease* includes the Lyme MSIDS questionnaire. An acronym for Multi Systemic Infectious Disease Syndrome, the term MSIDS gets to the root of how Horowitz wants us to think about this disease.

"It's based on a model of having seen twelve thousand people who say to me, 'I'm chronically ill. I don't know why I'm staying ill.'" Dr. Horowitz explained. "I found sixteen overlapping reasons why these people stay ill. Some of them are infections like Lyme, but there are many co-infections, viruses, immune dysfunction issues, allergies, inflammation issues—that's only to name a few—that are also keeping them sick. It's not just that they didn't treat the Lyme inflection properly; there are many other contributing factors to these patients' illnesses. Doctors aren't taking these factors into account, so they are calling it psychological: 'If I can't find the cause, then it must be in your head.'"

It's a simple idea, one that questions the way we think not only about Lyme but also about disease in general. If a tick has the capacity to carry many illnesses, why do we focus so heavily on only one? A very small percentage of Dr. Horowitz's patients are infected with only one tick-borne disease. So, of course, focusing on only one infection treats only one of the illnesses.

"The other issue in treating this disease is obvious. We have two standards for treating Lyme. One by the Infectious Disease Society of America, which says the blood tests are reliable, and the infection doesn't persist—it's cured after thirty days. Then we also have the International Lyme and Associated Diseases Society guidelines, which say the opposite: the blood tests are not reliable, and the disease can persist. This dichotomy makes the fifteen-minute HMO visit very difficult. Doctors don't have time to see if their patients have a multisystemic illness, and the perspective held by the IDSA means that they don't have to. We are all taught Pasteur's postulate in medical school, which tells us that there is one cause for one disease. Doctors don't think in terms of a multifactorial model, but there is an issue with that. If you go to a doctor with sixteen nails in your foot and complaining of foot pain, and only one or two of the nails are removed, you will still have pain. We have to look for all the nails. For me, that's really the key to understanding why people don't get better."

It seemed obvious to me. Having suffered from illness for so many years, the idea that only one thing could have caused that hardship was shortsighted to say the least. I wondered, though, how Dr. Horowitz expected people to respond to this theory. For years the mainstream medical community has emphasized the impossibility of Lyme persisting in the body after antibiotic treatment. What about this model was going to change their minds?

"The reason I think it will probably catch on and work is because it already has worked for so many people. I've seen twelve thousand chronically ill people in the last twenty-six years. My clinical experience is pretty broad at this point. Secondly, every chapter in my book detailing the sixteen-point model is heavily scientifically referenced. This isn't just my opinion. It's what the science is saying."

The scientific bias permeates all sides of this debate. Horowitz's studies might be completely refuted by Shapiro's or Ostfeld's, and vice versa. Just because the more mainstream science has government backing doesn't make it any more legit—the same could be said for Dr. Horowitz's work if his studies were backed by governmental institutions instead. I hoped, however, that faith in the stories of Horowitz's twelve thousand supposedly healed patients could help ground the conversation.

"The third reason I think this model can catch on," Dr. Horowitz continued, "is that our healthcare system right now is burdened by tremendous costs. We're basically going under, and not just from Lyme. There is an autism epidemic: one in eighty-eight kids are getting autism and no one knows why. There is a cancer epidemic. There is an Alzheimer's epidemic that is going to break the healthcare system by 2030. We don't have answers for these diseases, which are all, in a sense, at epidemic proportion, and no one is able to say why these people are sick. Right now, all we can do is throw chemotherapeutic drugs at them. We tell the autistic kids: 'We just don't know'; the Alzheimer's patients: 'Here, take Aricept and Namenda'; and the Lyme patients: 'You're cured.' That's not good enough. If people continue suffering, it's going to break the healthcare system financially. I think insurance companies will be very interested in a model that gets to the source of the problem."

Our conversation was about not only Lyme but also all of the conditions that shape the chronic Lyme experience. The term "chronic Lyme" is simply an umbrella for a number of different infections and imbalances in the body. Dr. Horowitz's mention of Alzheimer's and autism was very interesting to me, as he seemed to be referencing a common source for them. I knew a little bit about the connection with Lyme and Alzheimer's, but hadn't known of any possible connection to autism.

"Do you see a link between the illnesses you just cited?"

"Inflammation is the number one factor driving all of these diseases. Alzheimer's is inflammation of the brain. We know that environmental toxins getting into the body, mercury and lead for example, cause inflammation. Infections cause inflammation. Food sensitivities can cause inflammation. If you don't sleep well, that can even cause it. Many of the symptoms of Lyme: fatigue, joint pain, muscle pain, memory problems, mood disorders, are all also caused by these inflammatory molecules, and if you can lower the inflammation, people will feel better even if you haven't cured the disease."

I next asked him: "One of the things that seems to be the hardest to recover from is the psychological effect born from the treatment many patients receive at more mainstream medical institutions. Patients searching for answers may have heard twenty different responses from twenty different doctors. Can you speak to the effects of that?"

"Well sure. To be honest, most of the patients who come to me and have seen multiple doctors have heard at least once that their symptoms are all in their head. These people have PTSD just from seeing all these doctors and being told there is nothing wrong with them. They actually start to believe it after a while. They figure that doctors have reliable tests and they must know what they are doing. They figure the doctor knows better than they do. People have a very difficult time psychologically handling experiences like that.

"It is very hard for them to understand that psychology often plays a role in their illness, though it is likely not the cause. If a patient was slightly depressed and then was infected with Lyme and *Babesia*, that depression will get three times worse. Though the patient may have been depressed before, the main reason now they are so sick with these psychological symptoms is that the Lyme and the co-infections make it much worse. The more people are educated about Lyme and tick-borne [diseases], the more they will realize that these infections actually can cause psychological symptoms. If you treat the infections, your psychological symptoms should get better, assuming you don't have any other issues that have not been adequately dealt with. It's important to look at the mind-body connection. You can't just treat people physically; you need to look at all of the factors keeping them ill."

I repeated what he said, clarifying the idea to myself: "When someone previously suffers from psychological symptoms, the Lyme aggravates that." That simple idea was such a major player in my own experience, but it was still embarrassingly hard for me to wrap my head around. "Why is that? Is that an inflammation issue?"

"That's exactly what it is. Lyme causes inflammation; those same inflammatory molecules can cause mood changes. In the psychological literature, there is something called sickness syndrome. It's kind of like when you get the flu: you feel tired, achy, and moody, you want to withdraw. Technically, it's the inflammation that makes you moody, tired, and achy. When treating Lyme, if you take care to lower levels of inflammation in the body, patient mood disorders often get better. The problem with Lyme is that it mimics so many psychological diseases. We see people who have schizophrenic-like episodes. When we take them off their antipsychotics and give them antibiotics, all of a sudden they are no longer psychotic because they took an antibiotic. Lyme can cause psychological illnesses, as researched by Brian Fallon down at Columbia University. He is extensively published on those issues.

"It all comes back to the same idea for me," he continued. "This is multifactorial. Everyone has been looking for one cause for one illness, and they just aren't finding it. We are exposed to so much in the twenty-first century, so I believe we need to start looking at the Multi Systemic Infectious Disease Syndrome model, to look at all these other factors that may be causing illness. Let's apply it to every disease: Alzheimer's, autism, Lyme. I think it is going to be the answer for a lot of the chronic diseases we've seen in the twenty-first century. I sense that we are in the middle of a paradigm shift in medicine. I hope that the model I'm presenting can be a comprehensive model for many chronic inflammation diseases, not just for Lyme."

"And if there is any resistance to this model, where do you think that will come from? What do you think that will be driven by?"

"The resistance is mainly driven by the IDSA, which is holding the stance that Lyme is an easily diagnosable and curable condition. It's important to note, however, that when they did their double-blind placebo-controlled studies on the effects of antibiotic treatment, they were only looking at the effects of doxycycline and Rocephin, very simple protocols. When patients continued to display symptoms they claimed that meant antibiotics didn't work—but something more complex is going on there."

"If a patient has already been treated with Doxy and Rocephin and has failed the protocol, it's highly unlikely that giving it to them again is going to help them get better. This is the case for any infection. I will also note that none of the people who they tested in those studies had any co-infections, which almost every patient does have in my practice. Studying this disease requires a more complex perspective.

"To be honest, I think my model might allow the infectious disease doctors to realize that they can save face. I don't think they are wrong. I think that they are partially right, but that the conversation needs to get bigger. There is an autoimmune reaction in patients with persistent Lyme symptoms, absolutely no doubt. But the way many of these studies have been designed does not take into account the sixteen reasons that I've found are keeping patients ill.

"The mainstream doctors will be my number one opponents, but I think they will adopt this model of thinking once they realize it allows them out of the corner. They have trapped themselves in this place that says patients should be cured in thirty days and that's it. The insurance companies picked up on that. When they realize that it's time to look at chronic disease in a new way, I hope they will help fund further research for this treatment model to help prove it's effective. I already know it works for 90 to 95 percent of my patients. I need the best and the brightest of the scientists and the government to work with me now. I want to know what's wrong with the 7 percent of people I can't get better.

"We need to work together at this point to solve the problems of these chronic illnesses, not just Lyme. This is a model that requires us to stand and work together. We can't even do that for the most basic things. We can't allow kids to go hiking in the woods on school trips and not tell them there is a risk of Lyme and not check them for ticks. There are basic procedures that would prevent these healthcare costs, and we haven't even implemented those at this point."

"And why do you think that is?" I asked, my frustration barely muted by my attempt at professionalism. "What's behind that? Is there an advantage to not dealing with it?"

"No!" He matched my tone. "I think at this point everyone is overwhelmed with what's going on, and nothing has been integrated into one complete model. The government has to take the lead on this one. The

CDC needs to give guidelines to schools that say, If you're going to take your kids on a school trip and you're living in Lyme-endemic areas—truthfully, anywhere—have them do a tick check when they come back. Have their clothes sprayed with a tick repellent by the parents before they come to school. Know what are the symptoms of Lyme early on so that the children can be screened for it. It's [an] issue with pregnant women [too]. The OB-GYNs aren't screening women who come to their practice for Lyme, but the reality is that it can affect the fetus as it develops. When you realize how far the epidemic has really gone, it's shocking that these basic precautions have yet to be taken.

"What it will take is someone at a very high governmental level to admit that there's a major problem with the disease. The CDC just admitted that it is ten times worse than they suspected: it's not 30,000 new cases every year, it's 300,000. That doesn't even get the tip of the iceberg, if you look at the numbers: 0.3 percent of the American population were diagnosed in in 2012; that's over 900,000 people. That doesn't even take into account the people misdiagnosed with chronic fatigue, fibromyalgia, MS. If you take them into account, you probably have several million people per year diagnosed with this.

"We need everyone to sit down at the table and create a plan for ending this worldwide epidemic. Several years ago, the Chinese government told me up to 6 percent of their patients had been diagnosed with Lyme. I just met with the Health Minister of France, and she told me it had reached epidemic proportion across Europe. Outside of the United States, doctors are using the CDC treatment guidelines, so they are not using guidelines that are properly diagnosing and treating people. The CDC says themselves on their website that those guidelines are for epidemiological purposes. Doctors aren't supposed to use them for a clinical diagnosis, but doctors do. If we want to see change—we need to find another way to work the model."

PART IV

MAKING NOISE

Calvin took me to the planetarium for my twenty-third birthday. We'd been to the Natural History Museum countless times before, but I'd been to the planetarium only one other time, when we celebrated my eighteenth birthday—which came on the heels of my first and most devastating experience of neurological Lyme. On the previous visit, spending the day investing in worlds far away from my own, I felt proud to be where I was, engaging in ideas and conversations that I wouldn't have been able to understand just a few months before. I remember feeling larger than life on that trip. I held a place in space again. I felt huge.

On this more recent visit, though the venue was the same the experience could not have been more different. When the planetarium ceiling transformed into the night sky, instead of feeling I could reach up and touch it, I felt I was merely the size of a single atom. I was keenly aware of how many variables affect the course of our massive universe—and how it seemed nothing I did or thought would make the slightest bit of difference.

I have felt the same about tick-borne illnesses: that access to a healthy, fulfilled life post-infection was obtainable via only starry-eyed fantasy or the most gifted scientists—neither of which was coming my way. But I'm now starting to see glimmers of a new possibility for the world of Lyme disease, one where it's widely accepted as a complex, chronic illness that merits extensive study. I'm also realizing there might be a role for me to play in this world, an opportunity to help change the discourse of this disease—and even about chronic illness in general. Sitting still and silent isn't going to get us anywhere.

All those I've spoken with shared their stories for a reason. It's time to make some noise.

CHAPTER 25

A WEAKNESS OF THE WILL

To recap a bit: the Infectious Disease Association of America, the Centers for Disease Control, and much of the mainstream medical community continue to assert that the 10 to 20 percent of Lyme disease patients that present with persistent symptoms suffer from post-treatment Lyme syndrome, which is itself part of the phenomenon known as medically unexplained symptoms or functional somatic syndrome. Since they claim *Borrelia burgdorferi* cannot survive antibiotic treatment, any subsequent symptoms of Lyme must be attributed to "the aches and pains of daily living"[53]—not to active infection. "Somatic distress and medically unexplained symptoms have always been endemic to daily life," write Arthur Barsky and Jonathan Borus in their paper "Functional Somatic Syndromes." "The social and cultural characteristics of each era shape the expression, interpretation, and attribution of these symptoms. Thus, similar constellations of benign symptoms acquire different diagnostic labels and are attributed to different causes in different time periods."[53] In other words, there will always be individuals who feel illness without actually being ill. What they perceive is merely a product of their consciousness, whether their era chooses to dub the experience "Soldier's Disease," like in the Civil War era, or the more modern "chronic mono." Considered as such, they are more than just a medical phenomenon; they are also a social phenomenon.

That is one view of this issue, but there's another interpretation as well. What if chronic Lyme disease is not the most recent iteration of psychosomatic illness, but is actually part of another social phenomenon? There are a number of socially understood and accepted diseases that our society once dismissed exactly as it now dismisses tick-borne illness. Of these, AIDS and tuberculosis are perhaps the best known. But individuals suffering from lupus, MS, Parkinson's, even Crohn's disease have experienced—indeed, some still experience—the same silencing cultural pressures Lyme patients feel today. This is not a cultural anomaly; our society has consistently approached "mysterious" illnesses in the same manner, to the detriment of all sufferers.

Susan Sontag explores this idea in her book *Illness as Metaphor*. Focusing on the evolution of the social perceptions of disease, she offers insight into the significant consequences perception can have on patient narratives.

Sontag writes, "etymologically, *patient* means sufferer"—noting that the "suffering" of a typical patient does not represent the suffering we most deeply fear. We fear the "suffering that degrades," like from AIDS and polio, illnesses that "wither the body" to visually horrifying effect. This is one type of decomposition that inspires true fear, for both the sufferers and those witnessing the process. The degradation of the body and mind that occurs with chronic Lyme, however, is invisible to these witnesses. While some may notice changes in speech or memory patterns, the breaking down, the withering of the brain—as opposed to the withering of the body—is lost to them. Yet this invisibility doesn't keep patients of Lyme from falling victim to the same social fear as those of more obviously degrading diseases.

Sontag offers a possible explanation for this sort of pervasive fear: "Any disease that is treated as a mystery and acutely enough feared will be felt to be morally, if not literally, contagious."[55] It's a strange conundrum, blaming an uncomprehended illness on patients' morality or personality, as if it's something about their psychology or history that makes them ill.

However strange it may be, this is not a new phenomenon. In classic texts like *The Iliad* and *The Odyssey* illness appears as supernatural punishment. According to Sontag, this resulted from the Greek understanding of disease as being both "gratuitous and deserved."[56] Today, this Greek concept has evolved into our modern social conception of disease—disease as a product of will, or of character. When an illness is difficult to classify or understand, we don't always see its patients as victims; we see them as masters of their own fate. Sontag goes on to claim that the occasionally romantic idea of disease expressing character has been "invariably extended to assert that character causes the disease."[57]

Sontag suggests that patients with mysterious or unfamiliar illnesses, rather than being viewed as victims, are instead often considered cultural nuisances. Because the disease is strange and unknown, there is something strange and unknown about the sufferer as well. If we accept Sontag's claim that society views illness as a result of character, reflecting that claim back to chronic Lyme provides some interesting insights. The fact that the population of chronic Lyme sufferers is regularly dismissed by mainstream medicine suggests these patients are considered malingerers, even psychologically disturbed. As Sontag predicted, those dismissive adjectives describe and blame character, not infection or symptoms. And yet, these disparaging, marginalizing terms don't derive from the general population, something we can easily imagine; they derive from medical professionals, those we'd assume would seek scientific explanations for physiological symptoms.

A classic example of this phenomenon occurred in the 1980s, when no one understood why or how homosexual men were falling ill and dying from an enigmatic plague. Though it was not clear at first what specifically caused this deadly infection, the homosexual population was classified as the group spreading the disease. Because they suffered from a medical mystery, let alone because they were homosexual, early patients of what we now know to be HIV/AIDS were dismissed as social menaces, and as a result were denied for far too long the help they so desperately needed.

In 1978, when Sontag was writing *Illness as Metaphor*, cancer was still considered a mysterious disease; even though it is not contagious, cancer patients could feel as ostracized as AIDS patients did. "A surprisingly large number of people with cancer find themselves being shunned by relatives and friends and are the object of practices of decontamination by members of their household. Contact someone afflicted with cancer and it inevitably feels like a trespass, worse, like the violation of a taboo."[58] Though cancer patients did not have visible sores, and their disease did not seem to target one population—other than what was originally termed by some the "gay cancer"—they nonetheless felt ostracized by their society as a result of their sickness. Like Lyme patients, they too were the "thick-folder patients" doctors dreaded seeing in their offices. It didn't help that many suffered from ailments that likely resulted from "unsafe behaviors" like smoking or drinking: the only known causes of cancer at the time. Smoke, and you'll get lung cancer; drink, and you'll get cancer of the esophagus. Something about lifestyle, character, or "weakness of the will" was to blame. Indeed, cancer was considered deplorable until it was better understood; today it is fully accepted, the search for a cure regularly funded. Similarly, in the early 1900s multiple sclerosis was known as the "fakers disease"; today it is seen as a legitimate disease well worth eradicating.[59]

While the comparison of chronic Lyme to diseases like HIV/AIDS or cancer may seem a stretch, to me the above-described social and medical dismissal remarkably resembles that of chronic Lyme patients, and not just my own.

I read *Illness as Metaphor* in mid-2012, when I first started my senior project research. Along the way I cautiously wondered if Lyme disease might ultimately fit into the social patterns Sontag outlined. Through my experiences with both patient and doctor interviews, I can now say with confidence that it does. Lyme disease is another strong example of the "deplored" illness cycle: from social and medical dismissal all the way to ultimate acceptance and support. And though we may be in its worst stage, if history is our guide, in time we who experience chronic Lyme will start to receive acceptance and understanding of our suffering as well.

CHAPTER 26

REDUCING STIGMA

When I read Sontag's *Illness as Metaphor* in 2012 I was reading to better understand some of the motivations and psychological patterns underlying the negative experience of living with chronic Lyme. As I read I was reminded of some of my own encounters with the powerful urge, even compulsion, to keep my distance from sickness.

When I was about fifteen my parents took me to serve Thanksgiving dinner at a shelter for the homeless. The buffet trays of holiday fare looked pristine displayed on cloth-covered tables. I had set the dining tables as I would my own family's, taking care that the dinner knives faced inward, that the napkins folded over perfectly, their patterns complementing the tablecloth. But when we opened the door and commenced serving, for me the glory of the meal started to fade. Guests coughed into the potatoes and wiped their noses in the napkins. Many of them reached across the food to shake my hand in thanks, and I remember pulling away from them, disgusted. I knew my reaction was wrong. I was there to give thanks for life, but to me their sickness permeated the air. All I wanted to do was cover my mouth and leave.

Viewed objectively, it's a natural tendency to pull away from people who are sick, whether we do so consciously or subconsciously. Considered from a purely evolutionary perspective: prolonged proximity to the sick decreases our chances of passing on our genes, as many illnesses are contagious. Though many are not contagious, our instincts don't know that, and so we often treat the ill with disdain, working to maintain not just a physical distance but even a psychological distance in order to keep ourselves safe.

I am all too familiar with this tendency. My extensive experience with illness myself doesn't stop me from being scared by sick people, and I've often had to override strong impulses to pull away from others who are suffering. I remember finding this especially difficult during the summer after eighth grade. The clinic where I first received IV antibiotics was filled with pale, bony men; some could not speak, some struggled to walk. On my first day, I sat next to a man whose eyes were yellow, his arms black with bruises. I thought to myself, *I can't be this sick. I am not like this. I am not one of these people.* But six months later, the sick men I'd been scared of had become my friends. Once I was able to see them as human, and to understand them and their plight, my fear and disgust disappeared.

I was not the only person in that IV room aware of the effect public illness can have on its witnesses. Sitting for hours with needles in our hands and arms, I can't remember ever speaking about Lyme with the other patients at the clinic. Instead we filled the time talking about school, my siblings' sports games, or their children—anything but the disease that connected us. I imagine the reason for that omission concerned the fact that, out in the "real" world, we didn't want people to know we had Lyme disease, in case we'd be shunned by society or even dropped from our insurance.

A kind, patient man named Henry sat across from me each morning that summer. I remember one day he spent over an hour scrutinizing pages of thumbnails to help me pick my acting headshots. He'd regularly laugh and chat with my mom, as if he hoped their optimistic conversations would remind me of the beauty of life waiting outside. Henry worked on a farm about two hours from our clinic, and made the trip every day so he could heal and continue to provide for his family. As he was self-employed, he paid his own health insurance, but when his insurance company dropped him for being "over treated" for "post-treatment Lyme syndrome," he was forced to stop without a chance to say goodbye except by email. He closed his message saying he hoped we would both recover: but that even if he didn't, he was sure I would.

Societal opinions about Lyme negatively affect patient experiences every day, with industrial, medical, commercial, and social perceptions of illness constantly feeding off of each other. And though I hate to admit this, as much as I longed to see progress in the tick-borne disease dialogue, I believed I never would. Given the fear of speaking out I know from my own life, the polarizing biases introduced to me by Dr. Ostfeld and Dr. Keesing, and the rigid perspectives promoted by leaders like Dr. Shapiro, it seemed impossible I'd see progress in my own lifetime.

Though difficult hurdles in the medical and political spheres remain, I am starting to see strong potential for change at the personal level. I see power in one-on-one interactions and conversations, or emails and blog posts to a larger audiences. If, one person at a time, we can alter people's perspective about chronic Lyme, if we can help Lyme patients feel less dismissed, and then more accepted, that will help start to change social understanding of Lyme in general, broadening our cultural conception of the disease. The potential benefits of this progress are two-fold. The dismissal Lyme patients experience is often one of the hardest things to overcome in the healing process. With greater understanding among any one patient's immediate circle, and then broader circle, that patient will have a better chance of healing. And with greater understanding of the ramifications of chronic Lyme, more will be likely to voice their opinions about how harmful unchecked Lyme can be. When enough voices join the conversation, the medical and political spheres will eventually be required to act.

While I've been working to spread this message at the personal level, I've started to witness change at the medical level as well. One of the most promising comes from Ceres Nanosciences, a privately owned, technology-focused company. They are developing a proprietary particle technology called Nanotrap: a nanoparticle with a porous outer shell and an inner core containing chemical baits to attract certain cells and bacteria. Their most recent project, the Nanotrap High Sensitivity Lyme Antigen Test, uses this technology to directly measure Lyme antigens in urine. (An antigen is a "harmful substance that causes the body to produce antibodies."[60]) The test is said to be so specific it will end the subjectivity of Lyme blood testing.

I spoke with Mr. Ross Dunlap, the CEO of Ceres Nanosciences, about their work on this high-sensitivity test. Over the course of our conversation I felt tremendously hopeful that this new technology could be a game changer. If their development goes as planned, it wouldn't be just transformative at the individual level; their success would significantly bridge the gap in the chronic Lyme debate.

As it happens, Ceres Nanosciences did not set out to work on Lyme. Their original interest was in developing a diagnostic test for cancer. But, as Mr. Dunlap described, "a convergence of investors, scientists, and a large network of local supporters in Virginia, all with great interest in Lyme, coupled with our technology's maturation and application into other infectious disease areas, created the perfect opportunity to address a critical need for diagnosing Lyme." His company publically acknowledges that part of the need for this test is the incredible level of subjectivity and controversy that currently pervades the Lyme diagnosis.

That said, Dunlap stressed they have taken great care throughout the process to involve members of all sides of this debate, from renowned Lyme-literate doctors to influential medical professionals who deny the existence of chronic Lyme. "We want to help as many people as we can,"

Dunlap told me. "We're coming from a neutral place, working to under-stand the positions of everyone coming into this process, and also working to get to the bottom of what might really be going on with this disease."

The Nanotrap High Sensitivity Lyme Antigen Test looks for a specific lipoprotein found on the surface of only the *Borrelia burgdorferi* spiro-chete. A spirochete that's active in a mammalian host sheds this protein into the bloodstream; it can later be detected in urine. This means patients wouldn't have to wait for the immune system to catch up to the infection in order to test for Lyme; the test can detect infection as soon as the disease is active in the body.

One of Ceres Nanosciences's primary goals at the testing stage was to identify whether the *Borrelia burgdorferi*-specific lipoprotein is asso-ciated with only early-stage disease or if it is still present in patients with persistent and recurrent symptoms. Dunlap believes this objective in par-ticular—definitive answers regarding the persistence, or lack thereof, of the spirochete—is why so many from all sides of the debate have remained involved through the research process. "The Lyme-literate doctors want a better understanding of what's going on in their patients with persistent symptoms. And some of the other doctors are highly invested in disprov-ing the existence of chronic infection." Regardless of agenda, it is unique that both sides are working on one project, fusing their knowledge to de-velop a test that would finalize the debate one way or the other. Dunlap shared how every physician involved in this controversy wants a more reli-able blood test. And while these doctors weren't necessarily sitting togeth-er and sharing notes, they did work together through a private mediator. This alone was progress.

As for the preliminary results of their testing trial: so far, Ceres Na-nosciences has found that the *Borrelia burgdorferi* lipoprotein is present in the urine of patients in early stages of the disease. For patients thought to be suffering from later stages of Lyme, *patients presenting symptoms* show the antigen in their urine—even though they might test negative on a concurrent blood test, and even though they may have undergone years of antibiotic treatment. In fact, the urine test results in these latter cases—of patients with extensive antibiotic treatment—match the results of patients who've received much less antibiotic treatment. Again, the above concerns patients with active symptoms. From what Ceres has seen thus far, the antigen will show up during peaks of symptom recurrence, but it may not show during times of relative health. They do believe definitively that the antigen cannot show up in the urine sample unless the bacteria is *alive* in the system. Should that position hold true, positive results from this urine test could help prove that many chronic Lyme patients still suffer from active infection.

As for what's going on during periods of no symptoms: the assumption at this point is that the bacteria still exist in the body in cystic forms or other biofilm colonies—they are just dormant, burrowed in a manner we're not yet able to detect.

The test has been developed and the research is prepped for publication. The next step is to find hospitals and doctors to actually employ the test to further develop the research and results. As of September 2014, while Ceres Nanosciences was seeing a lot of interest from major East Coast hospital systems, Dunlap told me they had yet to find a hospital committed to running the test. It is only once the test has been integrated into a hospital's teaching division that they can work toward FDA approval, the last hurdle before the test being available to the public.

These results are still just preliminary. But even so, these developments offer multiple glimmers of hope for the chronic Lyme community. It's almost difficult to determine which of the following is better news: the possibility of proving persistent infection after antibiotic treatment, or the possibility of productive conversation between participants from both sides of the debate.

The living experience of chronic Lyme disease has been structured by an ideological fission that has had devastating effects on a shocking number of people. If there are 300,000 new known cases of Lyme being diagnosed every year, statistics suggests at least 30,000 new patients per year suffer from persistent symptoms. Could it finally be time to turn the corner for these patients? People like Horowitz and Dunlap suggest that it may be, but even that tremendous progress only concerns the medical side of the equation. chronic Lyme still suffers from its social stigma.

Returning to Susan Sontag's perspective, if Lyme disease is indeed in the midst of a "deplored" illness cycle, it is likely heading toward societal acceptance and support. Maybe so, but waiting for this cycle to run its course does nothing to help patients suffering today. And besides: who is "society" other than a larger collection of ourselves? If we think, speak, and write about the living experience of chronic Lyme disease in ways that perpetuate marginalization—if our language is overly biased, inaccurate, and dismissive—then we need to rethink the words we choose. To improve the experience of chronic Lyme, we need to ask ourselves, our families, our friends, and our government to rethink the way we speak about this disease.

CHAPTER 27

CASUALTIES IN THE WAR OF WORDS

Appendix C at the end of this book includes a chart comparing different Lyme disease "facts" cited by different sources: mainly the CDC and IDSA's "Ten Facts You Should Know About Lyme Disease"[61] and the "Quick Facts"[62] page of the International Lyme and Associated Diseases Society (ILADS) website.

Different sources will publish differing information to a certain extent. But we usually don't expect medical information to vary as much as it does between IDSA's "Ten Facts" and ILADS's "Quick Facts." In examining individual comparisons, in which sometimes one source completely contradicts the other, we see in word form the two sides of the chronic Lyme debate.

For example, the IDSA reports 70 to 80 percent of patients will see a bull's-eye rash, yet ILADS reports less than 50 percent of patients recall either a tick bite or a rash. The IDSA cites that anyone who has had symptoms for more than six weeks and has a negative blood test likely does not have Lyme disease; conversely, ILADS warns patients of the fifty-fifty probability of false negative test results. The IDSA states a few weeks of antibiotics will successfully treat most cases, whereas ILADS notes that short courses of antibiotics result in upwards of a 40-percent relapse rate.

Additional ILADS sources counter other statements on the IDSA "Ten Facts" list. While the IDSA claims the Lyme bacterium can be transmitted only through the bite of a tick, the ILADS Winter 2014 newsletter cites a study—an abstract of which was published in the 2014 January issue of the *Journal of Investigative Medicine*—suggesting that Lyme disease may be sexually transmitted:

> "Researchers tested semen samples and vaginal secretions from three groups of patients: control subjects without evidence of Lyme disease, random subjects who tested positive for Lyme disease, and married heterosexual couples engaging in unprotected sex who tested positive for the disease. As expected, all of the control subjects tested negative for Borrelia burgdorferi in semen samples or vaginal secretions. In contrast, all women with Lyme disease tested positive for Borrelia burgdorferi in vaginal secretions, while about half of the men with Lyme disease tested positive for the Lyme spirochete in semen samples. One of the heterosexual couples with Lyme disease showed identical strains of the Lyme spirochete in their genital secretions."[63]

These findings seem to refute the IDSA's claim that Lyme can be transmitted only through a tick bite.

In yet another example, the IDSA states that to infect a host the tick must be attached to the skin for thirty-six hours. Yet, in their article "What You Should Know About Lyme Disease," ILADS writes, "If [the tick is] infected, the spirochete is transmitted to the bloodstream of the person or animal during the bite."

Another concern is the timeliness of the data available. In the summer of 2013, the IDSA and CDC released an updated number of patients infected per year—300,000—which is ten times the number of patients cited in their Ten Facts list.[64] ILADS cites this figure on their site, adding that many patients of Lyme likely have yet to be diagnosed. I find it both curious and disturbing to note that, though both IDSA and CDC endorsed the revised figure, as of the end of 2014 IDSA has yet to reflect this change in their "Ten Facts You Should Know About Lyme Disease" document. In fact, this list, a resource for patients and doctors alike, has not been updated since May of 2011.

It seems the only item all parties can completely agree on is the IDSA's push to increase prevention of the disease.

It's problematic that both lists claim to be "facts." As many supposedly corresponding items exist in direct opposition to each other, many of these "facts" essentially cancel each other out. Each year, another 300,000 or more Americans will be diagnosed with this disease. Before they're diagnosed, many will likely seek guidance about their risk of infection, or their concerns about unusual symptoms they're experiencing. These individuals will either land on just one site or another—sites that would be either more helpful or less helpful, depending on your view—or they will land on multiple, contradictory sites, and will thus realize they must first pick a side before acting on any advice. They will need to choose, for example, if finding and removing a tick soon after being bitten will sufficiently protect them—following IDSA's statement that "to infect its host, a tick typically must be attached to the skin for at least thirty-six hours"—or whether it's much more likely that they were infected the moment they were bitten, as ILADS contends. These possible new cases will need to decide if not having found the bull's-eye rash can be trusted to indicate a corresponding lack of infection. New Lyme patients will need to choose whether they believe that a negative test result actually means they don't have Lyme, or whether they should pursue additional, perhaps even exhaustive testing in order to be sure. The ideological divide evidenced by these lists will negatively affect every individual in the ever-expanding patient body of tick-borne illnesses: currently cited as being thirty-four new cases of Lyme disease per hour in this country alone.

We are already seeing these negative effects play out. On the Lyme disease Frequently Asked Questions page of the CDC's patient resource website, a visitor asked: "If I have been diagnosed with Lyme disease, do I need to get tested for other tick-borne diseases (co-infections)?" The CDC reply begins, "Maybe. The blacklegged ticks that transmit Lyme disease can sometimes transmit babesiosis and anaplasmosis . . . ," but "the possibility of having three or more tick-borne infections or having pathogens such as *Bartonella* or Mycoplasma (which have not been shown to be tick-borne), is extremely unlikely." They also note, "There is a lot of misinformation regarding co-infections on the internet."[65]

The studies cited for this answer were all published in 2006. In the eight years since, all this information has been disproved. First, let's consider the statement "pathogens such as *Bartonella* or Mycoplasma . . . have not been shown to be tick-borne." Sources such as the National Center for Biotechnology Information[66] and the Columbia University Medical Center[67] have proven that both *Bartonella* and Mycoplasma are tick-borne bacteria. Second, though the reply includes babesiosis and anaplasmosis, it doesn't mention other common co-infections; one, *Ehrlichiosis*, regularly appears alongside Lyme. It's especially dangerous that the reply has not been updated to include the lethal Powassan encephalitis co-infection, which until 2013 was not believed to be present in the United States. Our earliest studies suggest there is a 10 to 15 percent fatality rate in reported cases of the Powassan virus.[68] The *New York Times* also noted that there is currently no treatment for this disease, which can leave nearly half of the victims it doesn't kill with "permanent neurological damage."[69]

Perhaps the most important misstatement in the CDC reply concerns the "extremely unlikely possibility" of having three or more tick-borne infections. Note the following, which appears in the Lyme disease portion of the NIH National Institute of Allergy and Infectious Diseases (NIAID) website, under "Co-Infections":

Ticks can become infected with more than one disease-causing microbe (called co-infection). Co-infection may be a potential problem for humans, because the Ixodes ticks that transmit *Borrelia burgdorferi*, the bacterium which causes Lyme disease, often carry and transmit other pathogens as well. A single tick could make a person sick with any one—or several—diseases at the same time. Possible co-infections include Lyme *borreliosis, anaplasmosis, babesiosis*, and *B. miyamotoi* infection.[70]

Many Lyme doctors today, including Dr. Horowitz and Dr. Raxlen, claim that almost all of their patients come in with more than one tick-borne infection. At the peak of my own illness, I was diagnosed with four tick-borne infections; my father was diagnosed with five. And almost every Lyme patient I interviewed had been diagnosed with two or more. Why is it that the information presented to new patients of Lyme—by the CDC, one of the most highly respected medical institutions in our country—does not reflect the current experience of dealing with this pervasive disease?

I'm also disturbed by the CDC statement: "There is a lot of misinformation regarding co-infections on the internet," as such conveys that all CDC guidance is definitive, comprehensive—to the exclusion of all other opinions. Given that CDC has not updated their site to reflect what is currently believed to be true information even by the mainstream establishment, in truth the "misinformation" of which CDC speaks derives from the CDC site itself, even from the very reply this statement appears in.

The CDC site altogether promotes an oversimplified perception of what it means to be diagnosed with Lyme, suggesting most of us are at risk of getting only one infection that can be easily diagnosed and treated. The reality of the situation, however, is that very few Lyme patients contend with merely one infection. chronic Lyme disease is often a series of complex infections that require a series of different antibiotics to treat.

Some of the viral infections—such as Powassan virus[71] and Bourbon virus[72]—successfully elude all known antibiotics.

I suggest that this disease operates within the multifactorial model that Dr. Horowitz and other doctors are now exploring. Without the premise that patients must fight multiple battles, it's no wonder so many are staying sick: they're being given only one of the many weapons they need to conquer their bacterial intruders.

So what would progress in this arena look like? What if institutions like the Centers for Disease Control, Food and Drug Administration, and Infectious Disease Association of America were to revise their stance on tick-borne illness, both internally and publically? What if the doctors whose work is currently thought controversial were instead celebrated for their pioneering development in this field? The body of evidence supporting the contrary stance grows larger every day; perhaps it's only a matter of time before it's deemed irrefutable. Yes, our medical system is reluctant to embrace change; indeed, it's practically founded on the stance that the only safe course is the conservative one. But history has proven the ability of much more entrenched entities to evolve—even to transform. I imagine we could see that happen in the Lyme world as well.

We don't have to look very far back into our history to find an analogous example. Consider the scourge of HIV/AIDS. In the first decade of the epidemic, the 1980s, so little was known about the human immunodeficiency virus that tens of thousands did not survive to see the publication of adequate treatment guidelines. (For example, the CDC issued guidelines for the treatment of pneumocystis pneumonia, then the most frequent cause of death among HIV/AIDS patients, in 1989. According to amfAR, The Foundation for AIDS Research, the U.S. year-end statistics for 1988 noted 82,362 reported cases of AIDS and 61,816 deaths.[73])

Until definitive information and the benefit of government backing was widely accessible, many doctors took it upon themselves to try to treat and prevent this deadly infection. Utilizing their knowledge of the body, of ill-ness, and of their patients, many moved out of the hospital system, opened private clinics, and practiced the medicine they believed appropriate at the time. Dr. Joseph Sonnabend, one of the first to notice the immune deficiency that would later be named AIDS, was one of these physicians.

A native South African, Dr. Sonnabend worked as a professor at Mount Sinai School of Medicine and with the New York City Depart-ment of Health until 1978, when he left to open his own private clinic for sexually transmitted diseases in Greenwich Village.[74] Without the back-ing of governmental or hospital institutions, Sonnabend conducted his own research on the then still unnamed syndrome. With the help of other physicians, he started the AIDS Medical Foundation to help fund his practice and research. Through his private clinic he treated thousands of early AIDS patients, working to develop his own treatment guidelines, many of which did not support or promote the commonly accepted opin-ions about the illness. He worked proactively and aggressively to treat the most lethal infections patients developed. He was also a strong patient advocate, known to publically criticize the mainstream medical commu-nity when he felt their medical decisions weren't in the best interest of his patients. Not surprisingly, though the infected community celebrated him, the mainstream medical community shunned him. His unconven-tional and controversial opinions on the treatment of HIV/AIDS even led to accusations of malpractice.[75] That is, until the CDC reconsidered their treatment guidelines and began to integrate his once-dismissed guide-lines into their own.

What is most notable about this story is that the mainstream medical community came to see the merits of—and eventually adopt—the beliefs of a smaller, highly controversial group of people. It was only once these two sides began working together that they were able to determine a more ef-fective course of treatment. And today, far from being considered a quack,

Dr. Sonnabend is thought to be one of the most important pioneering doctors in the early stages of the AIDS epidemic.

Sonnabend's experience with the mainstream medical community is almost identical to that of many Lyme-literate doctors (LLMDs). Forced to open private practices in order to treat their patients as they see fit, LLMDs are also often shunned by government institutions, refused funding, and accused of malpractice by insurance and governmental groups. Like Dr. Sonnabend, they act ahead of the curve of our burdened health care system, for which they are too often criticized and penalized.

If we look at the chronic Lyme debate with the history of HIV/AIDS in mind, perhaps we'll realize they tell the same story, that the only difference between the two sets of pioneering physicians concerns timing and numbers. When enough people are afflicted by a health menace, when the voices of those demanding change and acceptance grow too loud to be ignored: maybe that's when the obstacles to progress are finally forced to rethink their stances. I hold out hope that I may finally find that tidy ending I've always yearned for.

CHAPTER 28

ON ILLNESS, BELIEF, AND SPEAKING OUT

In *Far From the Tree* Andrew Solomon explores the concept of identity by investigating the lives of children who feel alien to their parents. As Solomon defines it, these children have "horizontal identities," or identities that are often considered flaws. They might be deaf, autistic, schizophrenic, or transgendered. Some suffer from Down syndrome, dwarfism, or other severe disabilities—while yet others are prodigies, or were conceived in rape. While most are children whom society regularly shuns, Solomon reveals how the immense love and devotion within their families help them forge powerful identities. Difference, in these cases, creates unity and strength.

Once the families featured in Solomon's book learned to overcome the traditional understanding of the words "healthy" and "normal," they found peace and understanding in all their relationships. Parents let go of expectations of what their children's lives were "supposed to be," and instead came to accept their eccentricities. They learned to appreciate their children for who they were, not who they expected them to be. "Horizontal identities" eventually became something comfortable, even positive.

I've started to think of chronic illness as another horizontal identity. Solomon writes, "The absence of words is the absence of intimacy,"[76] a sentiment that I imagine could also resonate with families affected by chronic disease. In my own experience of sickness, I too have felt starved for language. I've struggled to communicate my understanding of both health and sickness in my relationships and in my writing—perhaps because I have not yet owned one experience over the other.

A schizophrenic boy from *Far from the Tree* was instructed to post a self-mantra on his refrigerator, which meant he essentially revisited it several times a day. This single act changed the course of his treatment. It said, "I AM A GOOD PERSON AND OTHER PEOPLE THINK I'M GOOD, TOO."[77] This regular reminder of simple faith in himself, paired with others' faith in him, empowered him to get fully on board with his treatment plan, including bringing a more positive, productive energy to his therapy sessions. Belief in the validity and natural goodness of his life experience—of himself—turned him around.

Andrea Gibson, an artist and activist, also explores this idea in a piece entitled "On Illness, Belief, and Saying Yes." She writes: "Something I learned years ago in conversations with trauma survivors is [that] one of the most important things you can ever say to a person is 'I believe you.' I know the instances of my life where I have personally failed to do that have caused an overwhelming amount of pain."[78]

I consider these concepts in relation to my own life. If I had had cause to post, "I HAVE LYME DISEASE, AND I KNOW OTHER PEOPLE BELIEVE I DO, TOO" on my refrigerator years ago, would I have been more likely to speak with other Lyme patients about our experience? Owning the truth of my experience, and accepting the potential for others to see that truth, to even acknowledge that truth, could have helped me to see myself as part of a community. At the time I didn't believe a community of chronic Lyme patients even existed. I could not have been more wrong.

I'm still working to process, to own, all angles of my experience. It's been slow-going, as there is still so much to untangle. When I originally believed I had chronic Lyme, from which all my symptoms, physiological and psychological, derived, it all felt "fixable," the product of an infectious disease. But when the prestigious Boston medical community brought me to question the validity of chronic Lyme, the premise that I in fact suffered from mental illness felt so permanent, so unshakeable. Though I later returned to my initial belief, seeing Lyme disease as the primary culprit of my plaguing symptoms, I still suffer from the effects of that period of self-doubt. I also realize there's more to it than just the medical piece, that Susan Sontag's theories on the societal views of illness also contributed to my confusion, to my lack of feeling integrated. Between the various medical views of what I suffered, the variation among my symptoms and flare-ups, and the mixed, even shocking social response to my illness—it's no wonder I have yet to fully make sense of it all. The persistent whisper in the back of my mind that maybe I'm not yet healed, that I'll eventually present repeated, perhaps even new symptoms, only further complicates the problem. I hope that in time I'll be able to look back on this entire experience and find that no nagging doubts remain, that I've worked through the tangles and have properly wrapped up the experience as one that's behind me.

I know that my certainty about the physical reality of chronic Lyme disease will likely be seen as a classic example of "Post-Treatment Lyme Syndrome" patients, who desperately cling to anecdotes rather than to scientific "truth" in order to validate their stance. That's one way to read my experience. Though for a long time I feared being mocked or ridiculed for that very reason, I will not allow fear to silence me again. I have experienced and have witnessed the experiences of people whose lives have been ruined by a disease too often classified as an unexplainable phenomenon. Our experiences should not be pushed aside—considered unexplainable or unanswerable. Too many people suffer in remarkably similar ways for this "phenomenon" to be considered "unexplainable: case closed." We are not and cannot be satisfied by that lack of explanation. The real truth is that chronic Lyme merits a consideration of "not yet fully understood: studies pending."

I'm not a doctor or scientist. I don't conduct medical research, and I can't cite list of statistics or studies off the top of my head. I've developed my opinions and my worldview based exclusively on my life experience and the life experiences I've witnessed and been told about. I believe what I see in front of me, wholeheartedly. That said, I know that preaching my certainty won't change anything, and won't help anyone get better. What I can do—and what I hope will help others who suffer from this disease—is encourage people to speak out about the issues surrounding chronic Lyme and chronic illness in general. For now, should I be asked to choose sides in this polarized conversation, I will stand with the tick-borne disease community. But one day, I hope there will be no sides—that we all will find ourselves in the middle, figuring out the answers together.

For a long time I saw little hope for the future of chronic Lyme and its sufferers. I believed there'd always be some doctors willing to treat patients, but that they would remain the minority. I believed the health insurance juggernaut would ensure treatment was denied to thousands of sufferers—or else would cost them thousands of dollars out of their own pockets. And as a result, people like Melissa Edwards, or Ella McGovern, or Dave Riteman would remain sick for the rest of their lives. They would fall through the cracks—of the medical system, of society in general—paralyzed by assumptions about their experience rather than bolstered by the reality of what they actually suffer.

I no longer feel this hopeless: I see that the landscape is starting to change. More people seem willing to listen to the stories of Lyme sufferers, more physicians agree to hear their testimonies, and more scientists are working on their behalf. When I think about Susan Sontag's theory about the cycle of acceptance for illnesses like Lyme, I know that eventually the patients of chronic Lyme will be advocated for by the masses.

But some of us have less time than others. As of the end of 2014, Melissa and Zoe were still struggling with debilitating symptoms, unable to find, let alone afford, the treatment they desperately need. James Thomas's mother, Sarah, after shepherding her son through years of illness, was herself diagnosed with Lyme in April of 2013. My father experienced another relapse this fall, and returned to taking over ten pills a day. Every morning that I wake up with stiff knees or pain in my hands, I panic that I'm once again falling victim to tick-borne illness. And every day at least 1,132 people are added to the seemingly endless conveyor belt that is chronic Lyme.

I know that government processing is slow, that our hospitals and healthcare system are overburdened, that our doctors have limited time to spare: but I call on all who work within these systems to reconsider their stance on tick-borne illness. I ask that official treatment guidelines be updated to reflect the latest research on the persistent nature of this disease, and that legislation be passed that protects the physicians who treat chronic Lyme. I ask that doctors and hospitals embrace more objective and reliable testing options, and work together to push toward a less polarized treatment space. I ask all those who everyday are part of some system that affects Lyme disease to turn their thoughts to the hundreds of thousands of patients—and to think of them not as statistics, or anecdotes, but as people, as friends.

Yes, our current situation can be hard to navigate, but I believe that *awareness* about the crippling social and medical experience of Lyme—which even the CDC considers the fastest growing vector-borne disease in the United States[79]—should not be so hard to come by. Regardless of which side in the debate is right or wrong, hundreds of thousands of people currently suffer as the result of a tiny tick bite, and an even higher number of people have no conception of that suffering. It's time for that to change. Communication is the most powerful tool at our disposal. The more we speak out, the more we increase awareness, the more pressure we will create for change.

I was silent for a long time. I was terrified of sharing the truth of what happened to me because I feared how people would react. Though I was desperate to tell a story I felt completely certain about, my experience had been so plagued by subjectivity that such felt impossible.

Seventeen years have passed since my first Lyme diagnosis. Of those seventeen years, nearly nine of them have been spent sick. Of those nine years, eight have been spent so embarrassed and scared of my illness that I struggled to speak of it, even with members of my own family. I am incredibly relieved that my period of silence has passed, but I know very well how many others are still mired in their own silences. Almost every one of the Lyme patients I interviewed feared being identified as such. The disbelief in our experience—as well as the general stigma of illness—has so deeply permeated our social consciousness that some struggle to even name this disease out loud.

I have both witnessed and experienced the benefit of pushing through that fear and breaking that silence. With surprisingly few exceptions, when I share my story with others I see empathy on their faces. While the social dismissal of illness is real, and medical dismissal sometimes an even stronger force, I'm happy to report that on an individual scale empathy is not impossible to find. And as that empathy builds, as that one-on-one faith and understanding becomes stronger, I truly believe the living experience of chronic Lyme patients will improve.

For that, policy needs to change. Doctors need to treat. Tests need to be reliable. Full treatment needs to be available. And now that affordable health care is still a topic in the air, an unfinished story, insurance companies need to realize that, in the long run, it will be cheaper for them to let Lyme patients get the support they need from the beginning. In order for that to happen, however, the Lyme community needs the support of the public. We can earn that support by continuing to share our stories. With the power of words—spoken, written, posted, emailed—the narratives of the Lyme community can change the experience of future patients.

Every day I work to break my own silence, to share a little more about what it means to have lived with this disease, to have been treated by doctors in the way that I have. The more I share, the more faith I have in the power of that sharing. Our collective chronic Lyme voice is growing; before long it will be too loud to ignore.

For every disbeliever, I hope there will be at least one new believer. When they talk, I hope someone else hears them. I hope they too will want to share our stories, having learned something new about the way some of us move through this world. And for the first time, I think there might be a chance for what happens in my imagination to see itself leap into reality. I like to imagine this conversation as a new infection, an idea that is so contagious that once someone is exposed to it, they can't help but pass it along.

ACKNOWLEDGMENTS

To the team at North Atlantic Books, especially Erin, Tim, and Bevin—thank you for taking a chance on a senior thesis, and for your consistently thoughtful and patient feedback and guidance, which has helped transform this project into the piece it is today.

To Kirsten, my editor—thank you for spending your 2014 holiday season meticulously working through each page of this manuscript. Your work has helped make this a stronger, more potent piece of writing.

To Mary and Robert at Bard College—thank you for encouraging me to pursue a senior thesis on chronic Lyme disease and not on palimpsests, and then for encouraging me again to see potential in that project for something more.

To Michael at Bard College—thank you for guiding me through perhaps the most challenging phase of this project: its incarnation. You helped me to find my voice and realize that I had a story to tell.

To Dr. Raxlen—thank you for your trust, advocacy, and guidance in my moments of weakness and for being a part of this moment of strength.

To all of my friends and family—thank you for being there on the good days and the bad days, for celebrating my successes and helping me push through my setbacks. Special thanks to Erica for helping me make a big idea become reality.

To Calvin, Conor, Meg, Sean, Finn, Mom, and Dad—I could not have made it here without you. You are my biggest supporters and some of the most truly empathetic, strong, patient, kind, and loving people I know. You help me to learn from and find happiness in every experience: the good, the bad, and the ugly. I love you all more than you know.

And finally, to each and every person I interviewed for this project—your strength, knowledge, perspectives, and passions have forever changed the way I see the world. This is for you. Thank you.

APPENDIX A:
A BRIEF HISTORY OF LYME DISEASE

The following is a list of major events in the history of Lyme disease.

1909—Swedish dermatologist Arvid Afzellus presents a study about a "ring-like lesion" he observed in older women following the bite of a sheep tick. He named the lesion erythema migrans, what we now know as the bull's-eye rash.

1940s—German neurologist Alfred Bannwarth presents several cases of chronic lymphocytic meningitis and polyradiculoneuritis, some were accompanied by the erythema migrans skin legion.

1970s—A group of children and adults in Lyme, Connecticut, experience mysterious, debilitating symptoms. Two mothers in the community become patient advocates and start chronicling the experience of the sick people in their town.

1981—Dr. William Burgdorfer, while studying Rocky Mountain Spotted Fever (caused by tick bites) discovers that the Lyme spirochete, carried by ticks, causes Lyme disease. He is the first to discover the connection between the tick bite and the symptoms of Lyme disease.

1982—Medical community honors Dr. Burgdorfer's discovery and names the spirochete *Borrelia burgdorferi*.

1983—Research kicks off to better understand Lyme. The first record of Borrelia-like spirochetes is found on a neonatal blood smear.

1995—The Centers for Disease Control (CDC) reports 11,700 cases of Lyme in the United States.

2000—The Infectious Disease Society of America (IDSA) publishes treatment guidelines for Lyme disease.

APPENDIX A

2003—The International Lyme and Associated Diseases Society (ILADS) publishes their own treatment guidelines for Lyme disease.

2006—IDSA revises treatment guidelines for Lyme disease.

2009—CDC reports that there are 30,000 confirmed cases of Lyme disease in the United States.

2011—An autopsy of a 5,300-year-old mummy reveals *Borrelia burgdorferi* DNA.

2012—CDC names Lyme as one of the top ten notifiable diseases in the U.S.

2013—IDSA and CDC release an updated number of patients infected per year that was ten times the number of patients reported in 2009: 300,000.

APPENDIX B:
SAMPLE CHECKLIST OF SYMPTOMS

Each time I visited Dr. Raxlen, he gave me a checklist of symptoms to fill out. The following list is not comprehensive, and does not include symptoms of all tick-borne illnesses, but either I or someone I know has experienced every symptom listed below.

TICK BITE & RASH

❑ Rash may be circular with a raised center, shaped like a "bull's eye"

❑ Bite may be hot to the touch, raised

❑ Rash may disappear, and then return on another part of the body

HEAD & NECK

❑ Headache

❑ Neck pain

❑ Jaw pain

❑ Facial tingling

❑ Facial muscle twitching

❑ Spotty vision

❑ Double vision

❑ Itching / burning eyes

❑ Light sensitivity

EARS, NOSE & THROAT

❑ Sore / dry throat

❑ Dry mouth

❑ Pain in ears

❑ Sound sensitivity

❑ Consistent buzzing sound

❑ Consistent ringing sound

MUSCULOSKELETAL SYSTEM

❑ Joint pain

❑ Join inflammation

❑ Muscle pain / cramps

❑ Burning in hands and feet

❑ Weakness

DIGESTIVE SYSTEM

❑ Diarrhea

❑ New allergy development

❑ Extreme loss of appetite

❑ Unexplained weight loss or gain

REPRODUCTIVE SYSTEM

- ❑ Extreme menstrual pain
- ❑ Missed / irregular periods
- ❑ Difficulty getting pregnant
- ❑ Miscarriage
- ❑ Stillbirth

NEUROLOGICAL SYMPTOMS

- ❑ Unexplained tingling
- ❑ Unexplained numbness
- ❑ Burning sensations
- ❑ Consistent shaking
- ❑ Lightheadedness
- ❑ Dizziness
- ❑ Fainting
- ❑ Seizures
- ❑ Meningitis
- ❑ Irregular sleep patterns
- ❑ Memory loss
- ❑ Confusion
- ❑ Difficulty with speech
- ❑ Difficulty with writing
- ❑ Difficulty with reading
- ❑ Forgetfulness
- ❑ Encephalopathy (brain dysfunction)
- ❑ Encephalomyelitis (brain and spinal cord inflammation)

- ❑ Feeling as though you are "going crazy"
- ❑ "Brain fog"

OTHER

- ❑ Shortness of breath
- ❑ "Air hunger"
- ❑ Chest pain
- ❑ Night sweats
- ❑ Chills
- ❑ Cardiac issue
- ❑ Extreme fatigue
- ❑ Depression
- ❑ Anxiety
- ❑ Fever
- ❑ Immune dysfunction

APPENDIX C:

LYME DISEASE FACT CHART

Infectious Disease Society of America   **"Facts You Should Know About Lyme Disease"**   www.idsociety.org/Lyme_Facts   Last updated May 10, 2011
There were nearly 30,000 confirmed cases of Lyme disease in 2009 and more than 8,500 probable cases. The number has risen steadily since 1995, when there were only 11,700 confirmed cases.
To infect its host, a tick typically must be attached to the skin for at least 36 hours.
No information provided on mothers passing Lyme disease in utero.
No information provided on sexual transmission of Lyme disease.
Approximately 95% of all cases of Lyme disease occur in the Northeast and the Upper Midwest.
No information provided on the diversity of strains of *Borrelia burgdorferi*.
Anyone who has symptoms for longer than six weeks and who has never been treated with antibiotics is unlikely to have Lyme disease if the blood test is negative.
About 70–80% of people infected develop a red, circular "bull's-eye" rash, which shows up several days to weeks after the tick bite.
Most cases of Lyme disease are successfully treated with a few weeks of antibiotics.
Using antibiotics for a very long time (months or years) does not offer superior results and in fact can be dangerous, because it can cause potentially fatal complications.
No information provided on the long-term effects of Lyme disease.

International Lyme and Associated Diseases Society

"About Lyme: Making the Difference in the Diagnosis & Treatment of Lyme Disease"

www.ilads.org/lyme/lyme-quickfacts.php
Last updated March 2015

Lyme disease infects 300,000 people a year in the U.S.—10 times more than previously reported.
Fewer than 50% of patients with Lyme disease recall a tick bite.
Mothers can pass Lyme disease in utero.
Lyme may be sexually transmitted.
Up to 50% of ticks in Lyme-endemic areas are infected.
There are 5 subspecies of *Borrelia burgdorferi*, over 100 strains in the U.S., and 300 strains worldwide. This diversity is thought to contribute to its ability to evade the immune system and antibiotic therapy, leading to chronic infection.
The most common blood test, the ELISA screening test, misses 35% of culture-proven Lyme disease. Some studies indicate that up to 50% of patients tested for Lyme disease receive false negative results.
Fewer than 50% of patients with Lyme disease recall any rash.
There has never been a study demonstrating that 30 days of antibiotic treatment cures chronic Lyme disease. However, there is significant documentation demonstrating that short courses of antibiotic treatment fail to eradicate the Lyme spirochete. There are no tests available to prove that the organism is eradicated or that the patient is cured.
Short-term treatment courses have resulted in upwards of a 40% relapse rate, especially if treatment is delayed.
40% of Lyme patients end up with long-term health problems.

NOTES

1. Columbia University Medical Center, "Bartonella."

2. Melanie Reber, "Coinfections: A Synopsis."

3. Infectious Disease Society of America, "Statement for the House Foreign Affairs Committee Africa, Global Health and Human Rights Subcommittee's Hearing on Global Challenges in Diagnosing and Managing Lyme Disease—Closing Knowledge Gaps."

4. G. P. Wormser et al., "The Clinical Assessment, Treatment, and Prevention of Lyme Disease, Human Granulocytic Anaplasmosis, and Babesiosis: Clinical Practice Guidelines by the Infectious Diseases Society of America," 1115.

5. John Fallon, interview by the author, September 29, 2012.

6. Carolyn Welcome, interview by the author, July 30, 2013.

7. J. Feng et al., "An Optimized SYBR Green I/PI Assay for Rapid Viability Assessment and Antibiotic Susceptibility Testing for *Borrelia burgdorferi.*"

8. Merete Rietveld, "Mutant Bacteria and the Failure of Antibiotics, The Killers Within: The Deadly Rise of Drug-Resistant Bacteria by Michael Shnayerson and Mark J. Plotkin."

9. Eva Sapi et al., "Evaluation of In-vitro Antibiotic Susceptibility of Different Morphological Forms of Borrelia burgdorferi."

10. Columbia University Medical Center Lyme and Tick-Borne Diseases Research Center, "Persistence of Borrelia burgdorferi in Mice After Antibiotic Therapy."

11. D. F. Battafarano et al., "Chronic Septic Arthritis Caused by Borrelia burgdorferi."

12. V. Preac-Mursic et al., "First Isolation of Borrelia burgdorferi from an Iris Biopsy."

13. J. J. Nocton et al., "Detection of Borrelia burgdorferi DNA by Polymerase Chain Reaction in Synovial Fluid from Patients with Lyme Arthritis."

14. Nevena Zubcevik, "Better Diagnostic Tools Would Aid Fight."

15. Marianne Lavelle, "Mothers May Pass Lyme Disease to Children in the Womb."

16. Richard Horowitz's Facebook page, accessed September 10, 2014. https://www.facebook.com/drrichardhorowitz.

17. *Under Our Skin: The Untold Story of Lyme Disease*, directed by Andy A. Wilson.

18. Pamela Weintraub, *Cure Unknown: Inside the Lyme Epidemic*.

19. N. C., aka "Laura Williams" (name changed for anonymity), interview by the author, September 1, 2012.

20. John Ferro, "Where Foxes Thrive, Lyme Disease Doesn't."

21. State of New Hampshire Department of Health and Human Services Division of Public Health Services, "Tick Bites and Single-Dose Doxycycline as Prophylactic Treatment for Lyme Disease."

22. Kathleen McNerney, "Many Doctors Reluctant to Speak Publicly About Lyme Disease."

23. Fallon, interview by the author. See also LymeDisease.org, "News: Will Gov. Cuomo Sign or Veto NY Lyme Bill?"

24. Ibid.

25. Beth Daley, "Drawing the Lines in the Lyme Disease Battle."

26. LymeDisease.org, "News: House Passes Lyme Legislation; Now on to the Senate."

27. Fallon, interview by the author.

28. Alan MacDonald, "Hard Science on Lyme: Trials and Tribulations of Getting Borrelia Biofilms Accepted for Publication."

29. Jane Lerner, "Tick Secret Revealed: Westchester Researchers First to Prove Baby Got Babesiosis before Birth."

30. Denise Grady, "New Infection, Not Relapse, Brings Back Lyme Symptoms, Study Says."

31. Michael Specter, "The Lyme Wars."

32. Michael Specter, "'The Lyme Wars' That Tiny Ticks Have Wrought," interview by Terri Gross.

33. Pamela Weintraub, *Cure Unknown: Inside the Lyme Epidemic*.

34. Michael C. Carroll, *Lab 257: The Disturbing Story of the Government's Secret Plum Island Germ Laboratory*.

35. U.S. Department of Homeland Security, "Plum Island Animal Disease Center." As of January 2015, it appears that this statement has been removed from the DHS website; see also Robert Herriman, "Did Lyme Disease Originate Out of Plum Island?"

36. Robert Herriman, "Did Lyme Disease Originate Out of Plum Island?"

37. Infectious Disease Society of America, "Ten Facts You Should Know About Lyme Disease."

38. Brian Schwartz, "Lyme Disease Treatment."

39. John Jesitus, "Derms Slow to Embrace Subantimicrobial Dose Concept,"

40. Centers for Disease Control and Prevention, "Medicines for the Prevention of Malaria While Traveling: Doxycycline."

41. Johns Hopkins Bloomberg School of Public Health, "Lyme Disease Costs Up to $1.3 Billion Annually to Treat, Study Finds."

42. Andrew Solomon. *Far from the Tree: Parents, Children, and the Search for Identity*, 224.

43. Colin A. Walsh, "Pregnancy and Lyme Disease."

44. TAGS (Tick Alert Group Support), PO Box 95 Mona Vale NSW 1660, acccssed December 10, 2014, http://www.lowchensaustralia.com/pests/paralysis-tick/tick-alert-group-support.htm.

45. Section 504 of the Rehabilitation Act of 1973 works to ensure that children with a disability identified under the law attending United States elementary or secondary public schools receive necessary accommodations to help them succeed in the school environment "regardless of the nature or severity of the disability." This was intended to eliminate "discrimination on the bias of disability against students with disabilities" and to require school districts to provide "free appropriate public education" to each qualified student. To read more about Section 504, visit the US Department of Education website at http://www2.ed.gov/about/officies/list/ocr/504faq.html.

46. Dennis J. Bernstein, "Lyme Disease Is a Feminist Issue: An Interview with Sini Anderson."

47. D. E. Hoffman and A. J. Tarzanian, "The Girl Who Cried Pain: A Bias Against Women in the Treatment of Pain."

48. Laurie Edwards, "The Gender Gap in Pain."

49. Liz Szabo, "Women Less Likely to Get Immediate Heart Attack Treatment."

50. Simon Hatcher and Bruce Arroll, "Assessment and Management of Medically Unexplained Symptoms," 1124.

51. A. L. Hassett et al., "Psychiatric Comorbidity and Other Psychological Factors in Patients with 'Chronic Lyme Disease,'" 607.

52. A. J. Barsky and J. F. Borus. "Functional Somatic Syndromes," 910.

53. Wormser et al., "The Clinical Assessment, Treatment, and Prevention of Lyme Disease, Human Granulocytic Anaplasmosis, and Babesiosis," 1115.

54. Barsky and Borus, "Functional Somatic Syndromes," 911.

55. Susan Sontag, *Illness as Metaphor and AIDS and Its Metaphors*, 6.

56. Ibid., 43.

57. Ibid., 44.

58. Ibid., 6.

59. Ibid., 113.

60. Merriam-Webster, "Antigen."

61. Infectious Disease Society of America, "Ten Facts You Should Know About Lyme Disease."

62. International Lyme and Associated Diseases Society, "ILADS About Lyme: Making the Difference in the Diagnosis and Treatment of Lyme Disease."

63. Guinnevere Stevens, "Lyme Disease May Be Sexually Transmitted, Study Suggests."

64. Centers for Disease Control and Prevention, "CDC Provides Estimate of Americans Diagnosed with Lyme Disease Each Year."

65. Centers for Disease Control and Prevention, "Lyme Disease Frequently Asked Questions (FAQ)."

66. R. C. Bransfield, "The Psychoimmunology of Lyme/Tick-Borne Diseases and Its Association with Neuropsychatric Symptoms."

67. Ibid.

68. Alan P. Dupis et al., "Black-Legged Ticks Linked to Encephalitis in New York State."

69. *New York Times* Editorial Board, "Dangerous Ticks."

70. National Institute of Allergy and Infectious Diseases, "Lyme Disease."

71. Centers for Disease Control and Prevention, "Frequently Asked Questions."

72. University of Kansas Hospital, "New 'Bourbon Virus' Linked to Death."

73. AmfAR, "Thirty Years of HIV/AIDS: Snapshots of an Epidemic."

74. Bruce Nussbaum. *Good Intentions: How Big Business and the Medical Establishment Are Corrupting the Fight Against AIDS.*

75. Sean Strub, "The Good Doctor."

76. Solomon, *Far from the Tree,* 5.

77. Ibid., 325.

78. Andra Gibson, "On Illness, Belief, and Saying Yes."

79. International Lyme and Associated Diseases Society, "ILADS About Lyme."

WORKS CITED

AmfAR. "Thirty Years of HIV/AIDS: Snapshots of an Epidemic." Acessed February 4, 2015. http://amfar.org/thirty-years-of-hiv/aids-snapshots-of-an-epidemic.

Barsky, A. J., and J. F. Borus. "Functional Somatic Syndromes." *Annals of Internal Medicine* 130, no. 11 (June 1999): 910–21.

Battafarano, D. F., J. A. Combs, R. J. Enzenauer, and J. E. Fizpatrick. "Chronic Septic Arthritis Caused by Borrelia burgdorferi." *Clinical Orthopaedics and Related Research* 297 (December 1993): 238–41.

Bernstein, Dennis J. "Lyme Disease Is a Feminist Issue: An Interview with Sini Anderson." *Truthout.* June 19, 2004. http://truth-out.org/news/item/24405-lyme-disease-is-a-feminist-issue-an-interview-with-sini-anderson.

Bransfield, R. C. "The Psychoimmunology of Lyme/Tick-Borne Diseases and Its Association with Neuropsychiatric Symptoms." *The Open Neurology Journal* 6 (2012): 88–93. http://www.ncbi.nlm.nih.gov/pmc/articles/PMC3474947.

Carroll, Michael C. *Lab 257: The Disturbing Story of the Government's Secret Plum Island Germ Laboratory.* New York: William Morrow, 2004.

Centers for Disease Control and Prevention. "CDC Provides Estimate of Americans Diagnosed with Lyme Disease Each Year." August 19, 2013. http://www.cdc.gov/media/releases/2013/p0819-lyme-disease.html.

———. "Frequently Asked Questions." Last modified February 9, 2015. http://ww.cdc.gov/powassan/faqs.html.

———. "Lyme Disease Frequently Asked Questions (FAQ)." Last modified March 4, 2015. http://cdc.gov/lyme/faq.

———. "Medicines for the Prevention of Malaria While Traveling: Doxycycline." Accessed February 8, 2015. http://www.cdc.gov/malaria/resources/pdf/fsp/drugs/doxycycline.pdf.

Columbia University Medical Center Lyme and Tick-Borne Diseases Rearch Center. "Bartonella." Accessed February 8, 2015. http://columbia-lyme.org/patients/tbd_bartonella.html.

———. "Persistence of Borrelia Burgdorferi in Mice after Antibiotic Therapy." Accessed January 7, 2015. http://columbia-lyme.org/research/keyarticles.html.

Daley, Beth. "Drawing the Lines in the Lyme Disease Battle." *Boston Globe.* June 2, 2013. http://www.bostonglobe.com/metro/2013/06/01/lyme-disease-rise-and-controversy-over-how-sick-makes-patients/OT4rCTy9qRYh25GsTocBhL

/story.html.

Dupis, Alan P., Ryan J. Peters, Melissa A. Prusinski, Richard C. Falco, Richard S. Ost-feld, and Laura D. Kramer. "Black-Legged Ticks Linked to Encephalitis in New York State." *Cary Institute of Ecosystem Studies.* July 15, 2013. http://www.cary-institute.org/newsroom/black-legged-ticks-linked- encephalitis-new-york-state.

Edwards, Laurie. "The Gender Gap in Pain." *New York Times,* March 16, 2003. http://www.nytimes.com/2013/03/17/opinion/sunday/women-and-the-treat-ment-of-pain.html?_r=0

Feng J., T. Wang, S. Zhang, W. Shi, and Y. Zhang. "An Optimized SYBR Green I/PI Assay for Rapid Viability Assessment and Antibiotic Susceptibility Testing for Borrelia burgdorferi." *PLoS ONE* 9, no. 11 (November 3, 2013).

Ferro, John. "Where Foxes Thrive, Lyme Disease Doesn't." *Poughkeepsie Journal,* September 20, 2012. http://poughkeepsiejournal.com/story/news/health/lyme-disease/2014/03/20/lyme-foxes/6657687.

Gibson, Andrea. "On Illness, Belief, and Saying Yes." *The Body Is Not an Apology* (blog). July 24, 2014. http://thebodyisnotanapology.tumblr.com/post/92737802410/on-illness-belief-and-saying-yes.

Grady, Denise. "New Infection, Not Relapse, Brings Back Lyme Symptoms, Study Says." *New York Times.* November 14, 2012, A22.

Hassett, A. L., D. C. Radvanski, S. Buyske, S. V. Savage, and L. H. Sigal. "Psychiatric Comorbidity and Other Psychological Factors in Patients with 'Chronic Lyme Disease.'" *American Journal of Medicine* 122, no. 9 (September 2009): 843–50.

Hatcher, Simon, and Bruce Arroll. "Assessment and Management of Medically Unex-plained Symptoms." *British Medical Journal* 336 (2008): 1124–28. http://www.ncbi.nlm.nih.gov/pmc/articles/PMC2386650/

Herriman, Robert. "Did Lyme Originate out of Plum Island?" *Examiner,* October 30, 2010. http://examiner.com/article/did-lyme-disease-originate-out-of-plum-island.

Hoffman, D. E., and A. J. Tarzian. "The Girl Who Cried Pain: A Bias Against Wom-en in the Treatment of Pain." *Journal of Law, Medicine, and Ethics* 29, no. 1 (Spring 2001): 13–27. http://www.forgrace.org/documents/hoffmann.pdf

Horowitz, Richard. (2014, September 10). "I have had women who have had mul-tiple miscarriages... Contemporary Ob/Gyn 35:48-64." *Facebook.*

Infectious Disease Society of America. "Global Health and Human Rights Subcom-mittee's Hearing on Global Challenges in Diagnosing and Managing Lyme Dis-ease—Closing Knowledge Gaps Submitted by the Infectious Diseases Society of America." Statement presented for the House Foreign Affairs Committee. July 17, 2012.

———. "Ten Facts You Should Know About Lyme Disease." Last modified May 20, 2011. http://idsociety.org/Lyme_Facts.

International Lyme and Associated Diseases Society. "ILADS About Lyme: Making the Difference in the Diagnosis and Treatment of Lyme Disease. Accessed February 4, 2015. http://ilads.org/lyme/lyme-quickfacts.php.

———."Lyme Disease May Be Sexually Transmitted, Study Suggests." *ILADS News: International Lyme and Associated Diseases Society* 7 (Winter 2014).

Jesitus, John. "Derms Slow to Embrace Subantimicrobial Dose Concept." *Dermatology Times.* February 1, 2014. http://dermatologytimes.modernmedicine.com /dermatology-times/content/tags/acne-treatment/derms-slow-embrace-subanti-microbial-dose-concept?page=full.

Johns Hopkins Bloomberg School of Public Health. "Lyme Disease Costs Up to $1.3 Billion Annually to Treat, Study Finds." *Infection Control Today.* February 5, 2015. http://www.infectioncontroltoday.com/news/2015/02/lyme-disease -costs-up-to-13-billion-annually-to-treat-study-finds.aspx.

Lavelle, Marianne. "Mothers May Pass Lyme Disease to Children in the Womb." *Scientific American,* September 22, 2014. http://scientificamerican.com/article /mothers-may-pass-lyme-disease-to-children-in-the-womb.

Lerner, Jane. "Tick Secret Revealed: Westchester Researchers First to Prove Baby Got Babesiosis before Birth." LoHud.com. July 6, 2012. http://archive.lohud .com/article/20120706/NEWS02/307060050/Tick-secret-revealed-Westches-ter-researchers-first-prove-baby-got-babesiosis-before-birth.

LymeDisease.org. "News: House Passes Lyme Legislation; Now on to the Senate." September 9, 2014. http://lymedisease.org/news/lyme_disease_views/house -passes-lyme-bill.html.

———. "News: Will Gov. Cuomo Sign or Veto NY Lyme Bill?" July 9, 2014. http:// lymedisease.org/news/lyme_disease_views/will-cuomo-sign-lyme-bill.html.

MacDonald, Alan. "Hard Science on Lyme: Trials and Tribulations of Getting Borrelia Biofilms Accepted for Publication." August 2, 2013. http://lymedisease .org/news/hardscienceonlyme/the-rest-of-the-story-trials-and-tribulations-of -getting-borrelia-biofilms-acccepted-for-publication.html.

McNerney, Kathleen. "Many Doctors Reluctant to Speak Publicly About Lyme Disease." *WBUR's Common Health: Reform and Reality.* June 29, 2012. http://com-monhealth.wbur.org/2012/06/doctors-lyme-disease.

Merriam-Webster. "Antigen." Accesssed December 29, 2014. http://www.merriam -webster.com/dictionary/antigen.

National Institute of Allergy and Infectious Diseases. "Lyme Disease." Accessed February 4, 2015. http://www.niaid.nih.gov/topics/lymeDisease/research/Pages/co

-infection.aspx

New York Times Editorial Board. "Dangerous Ticks." *New York Times.* August 27, 2013, A20. http://www.nytimes.com/2013/08/27/opinion/dangerous-ticks .html?_r=0.

Nocton, J. J., F. Dressler, B. J. Rutledge, P. N. Rys, D. H. Persing, and A. C. Steere. "Detection of Borrelia burgdorferi DNA by Polymerase Chain Reaction in Synovial Fluid from Patients with Lyme Arthritis." *New England Journal of Medicine,* 330, no. 4 (January 1994): 229–34.

Nussbaum, Bruce. *Good Intentions: How Big Business and the Medical Establishment Are Corrupting the Fight Against AIDS.* New York: Atlantic Monthly Press, 1990.

Preac-Mursic, V., H. W. Pfister, H. Spiegel, R. Burk, B. Wilske, S. Reinhardt, and R. Böhmer. "First Isolation of Borrelia burgdorferi from an Iris Biopsy. *Journal of Clinical Neuro-Ophthalmology* 13, no. 3 (September 1993): 155–61.

Reber, Melanie. "Coinfections: A Synopsis." *Lyme Info.* Last modified January 2005. http://lymeinfo.net/coinfectionarticle.html.

Rietveld, Merete. "Mutant Bacteria and the Failure of Antibiotics, The Killers Within: The Deadly Rise of Drug-Resistant Bacteria by Michael Shnayerson and Mark J. Plotkin." *Genome News Network.* April 4, 2003. http://www.genomenewsnetwork.org/articles/04_03/killers_rev.php.

Sapi, Eva, Navroop Kaur, Samuel Anyanwu, David F. Luecke, Akshita Datar, Seema Patel, and Michael Rossi and Raphael B. Stricker. "Evaluation of In-vitro Antibiotic Susceptibility of Different Morphological Forms of Borrelia burgdorferi." *Journal of Infection and Drug Resistance* 4 (2011): 97–113.

Schwartz, Brian. "Lyme Disease Treatment." *Johns Hopkins Arthritis Center.* Last modified October 10, 2012. http://www.hopkinsarthritis.org/arthritis-info /lyme-disease/lyme-disease-treatment.

Solomon, Andrew. *Far from the Tree: Parents, Children, and the Search for Identity.* New York: Scribner, 2012.

Sontag, Susan. *Illness as Metaphor and AIDS and Its Metaphors.* New York: Picador USA, 1990.

Specter, Michael. "The Lyme Wars." *The New Yorker.* July 1, 2013.

———. "'The Lyme Wars' That Tiny Ticks Have Wrought." Interview by Terri Gross. *Fresh Air.* NPR. July 26, 2013. http://www.wbur.org/npr/195223507 /the-lyme-wars-that-tiny-ticks-have-wrought.

State of New Hampshire Department of Health and Human Services Division of Public Health Services. "Tick Bites and Single-Dose Doxycycline as Prophylactic Treatment for Lyme Disease." ManchesterNH.gov. Accessed February 8, 2015.

http://www.manchesternh.gov/portals/2/Departments/health/Prophylaxis%20 following%20tick%20bites.pdf.

Strub, Sean. "The Good Doctor." *POZ: Health, Life, & HIV.* July 1998.

Szabo, Liz. "Women Less Likely to Get Immediate Heart Attack Treatment." *USA Today.* February 21, 2012.

Under Our Skin: The Untold Story of Lyme Disease. Andy A. Wilson, director. Open Eye Pictures Inc., 2009.

University of Kansas Hospital. "New 'Bourbon Virus' Linked to Death." *Medical News Network.* Accessed February 4, 2015. http://medicalnewsnetwork.org /newsnetwork/doctalk/b?bourbonvirus.

U. S. Department of Homeland Security. "Plum Island Animal Disease Center." *Science and Technology Directorate.* October 6, 2013. http:// www.dhs.gov/st-piadc.

Walsh, Colin A. "Pregnancy and Lyme Disease." Lecture presented at the International Lyme and Associated Disease Society Annual Scientific Meeting, Cambridge, UK. October 2007.

Winetraub, Pamela. *Cure Unknown: Inside the Lyme Epidemic.* New York: St. Martin's Griffin, 2009.

Wormser, G. P., R. J. Dattwyler, E. D. Shapiro, J. J. Halperin, A. C. Steere, M. S. Klempner, and P. J. Krause, et al. "The Clinical Assessment, Treatment, and Prevention of Lyme Disease, Human Granulocytic Anaplasmosis, and Babesiosis: Clinical Practice Guidelines by the Infectious Diseases Society of America." *Clinical Infectious Diseases* 43, no. 9 (November 2006): 1089–134.

Zubcevik, Nevena. "Better Diagnostic Tools Would Aid Fight." *Poughkeepsie Journal,* June 28, 2013. http://www.poughkeepsiejournal.com/story/opinion/columnists/2014/03/26/lyme-nevena-zubcevik/6918305.

ABOUT THE AUTHOR

Allie Cashel was first diagnosed with Lyme disease in June of 1998; she has been a sufferer of Lyme, Babesiosis, Ehricliosis, and Bartonellosis for seventeen years. While studying at Bard College, she conducted a series of interviews with chronic Lyme patients in New York and around the world, revealing a complex world of suffering within the Lyme community. Cashel now works as a passionate advocate for increased awareness of Lyme disease and other chronic illnesses: she is on the Junior Board of the Global Lyme Alliance, guest lectures at Bard College about her work, and has created the online community "Suffering the Silence" to build awareness around Lyme and other chronic illnesses. (Visit sufferingthesilence .com for more information.) She currently lives in New York City with her boyfriend, Calvin, and her dog, Percy.

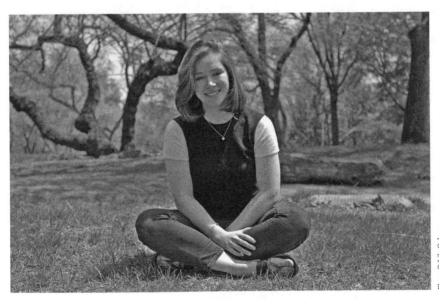

Photo © Lily Colman